Society, Environment and Statistics

This interdisciplinary book series demonstrates the significance of statistical science in quantifying and understanding societal and environmental changes, while effectively managing resources. The series invites manuscripts that cover a wide range of themes, including original research in traditional fields, emerging topics, practical applications, and connections between novel findings and established works. Particularly encouraged are submissions that showcase methodologies, case studies, good practices and innovative solutions addressing the complex challenges of the United Nations' Sustainable Development Goals (SDGs). Rigorously peer-reviewed, all contributions adhere to the highest standards of scientific literature.

Andrea Bellavia

Statistical Methods for Environmental Mixtures

A Primer in Environmental Epidemiology

Springer

Andrea Bellavia
Department of Medicine
Harvard Medical School
Boston, MA, USA

ISSN 2948-2763 ISSN 2948-2771 (electronic)
Society, Environment and Statistics
ISBN 978-3-031-78986-1 ISBN 978-3-031-78987-8 (eBook)
https://doi.org/10.1007/978-3-031-78987-8

This Springer imprint is published by the registered company Springer Nature Switzerland AG
The registered company address is: Gewerbestrasse 11, 6330 Cham, Switzerland

Preface

Environmental toxicants such as pollutants, metals, and chemical compounds are ubiquitous in our modern world. Humans are exposed to hundreds of potentially harmful substances, which are found as environmental mixtures in everyday sources of exposures from the living environment to consumer products. These complex exposures can affect human health through a variety of biological mechanisms, presenting a substantial challenge to public health. Epidemiologic studies attempting to assess the health effects of environmental mixtures have to take into account this complex exposure definition as a combined group of multiple factors, which poses considerable challenges from an analytical perspective. Over the last decade, substantial research efforts have been made toward the clarification of these challenges and the development and application of statistical methodologies that can incorporate the complexity of environmental mixtures in population-based studies.

The goal of this book is to provide an introduction to the statistical framework for assessing mixture-health associations in environmental epidemiology. This introductory tool is aimed at students and researchers in epidemiology who are interested in integrating environmental mixtures in the design and analysis of population-based studies. As such, the focus is kept on methods interpretation and application rather than on technical mathematical and computational details. The core message of the book, on which the selection of topics and the presentation format is based, is that a comprehensive assessment of mixture-health associations should adopt a triangulated approach where several methods are evaluated and presented. To such end, for all chapters, particular emphasis is given on the advantages and limitations of each approach, and the specific contribution they can provide to the research questions of interest.

The number of statistical approaches that have been suggested as potential methods for mixture studies is considerably high. The goal of this primer is not to list and discuss all these potential approaches, but rather to provide a summary introduction to different classes of methods, their different goals and perspectives, and how they can be used to complement each other in practical applications. Within each chapter, details and illustration are provided for selected methodologies that have achieved an established appreciation within the field, while additional references are provided for alternative techniques that can be considered on a case-by-case basis. This selection should not be read as a discrimination between better and worse approaches. Presented methods were rather selected based on specific features that facilitate their potential implementation in routine analyses, including the availability of documented software material; the existence of several illustrations and applications in applied settings of different complexity; their robustness and validity as documented by published methodological review and comparison papers. As discussed in the final chapter, the analytical tools discussed in this book provide a basic yet comprehensive set of approaches that can be used to design and conduct a rigorous analytical plan for assessing mixture-health effects in epidemiologic studies. All methods presented can be implemented in the R statistical software, and are often accompanied by exceptional user-friendly vignettes and tutorials developed by the authors. To facilitate implementation of these approaches, I have included in an accompanying web page (https://github.com/andreabellavia/statsmixtures) some basic R code to replicate the analysis of a simulated dataset included as illustrative example in this book, together with link to publicly available software material for the discussed methodologies.

There are several people I'd like to thank. This book is an extension of the class material for the graduate course on this topic that I have been teaching at the Harvard T.H. Chan School of Public Health since 2018. The course would not have happened without the help and support of Russ Hauser, who encouraged me to design a novel course on a topic that, at that time, was still unfamiliar and mysterious to many. Most of what I have learned in environmental statistics is the fruit of the exceptional mentoring of Paige L. Williams and of the several insightful conversations with Brent Coull. I am also grateful for the mentoring of Tamarra James-Todd, Andrea Baccarelli, and Marc Weisskopf, who introduced me to the world of environmental epidemiology. A special thanks also goes to my longtime friends and colleagues Stefano Renzetti and Ran Rotem, for the engaging conversations on the topics of this book and for their insightful comments on a preliminary version of the text. Last but not least, thanks to Marlee R. Quinn for her love and support throughout the process and for the precious help with the writing of this book.

Boston, MA, USA Andrea Bellavia
September 2024

Contents

1 Environmental Mixtures 1
1.1 Environmental Mixtures Within the Exposome Framework 1
1.2 Mixtures Assessment in Environmental Epidemiology 2
1.3 Questions of Interest in Mixtures Research 3
1.4 Structure of the Book 4
1.5 Illustrative Example and Software Material 5
References 6

2 Characterizing Environmental Mixtures 9
2.1 Overview of Unsupervised Analyses for Environmental Mixtures 9
2.2 Data Preprocessing 10
2.3 Correlation Analysis 13
2.3.1 Correlation Network Analysis 16
2.4 Principal Component Analysis: (PCA) 17
2.4.1 Principal Components Derivation 17
2.4.2 Choosing the Number of Components 19
2.4.3 Making Sense of Component Interpretation 20
2.4.4 PCA: Concluding Remarks 21
References 22

3 Regression-Based Approaches for Mixture-Health Associations 25
3.1 Overview of Regression Modeling in Environmental Mixtures Research 25
3.2 Classical Regression Approaches and Their Limitations 26
3.2.1 Environmental-Wide Association Studies 26
3.2.2 Co-confounding Between Mixture Components 26
3.2.3 Multiple Regression 28
3.2.4 Multicollinearity 29
3.3 Penalized Regression 31
3.3.1 Bias-Variance Trade-Off 31
3.3.2 Ridge 33
3.3.3 LASSO 35

3.3.4 Elastic Net 36
3.3.5 Practical Notes and Relevant Extensions 38
3.4 Penalized Regression: Concluding Remarks 39
References 40

4 Mixture Indexing Approaches 43
4.1 Introduction to Indexing 43
4.2 Unsupervised Summary Scores 45
4.3 Weighted Quantile Sum (WQS) Regression 46
4.3.1 Estimation 47
4.3.2 Results Interpretations and Practical Considerations 48
4.3.3 Extensions of the WQS Framework 49
4.3.4 Quantile G-computation 51
4.3.5 WQS: Concluding Remarks 53
4.4 Alternative Supervised Approaches 54
References 55

5 Flexible Approaches for Complex Settings 59
5.1 Assumptions of Linearity and Additivity in Regression Modeling 59
5.1.1 Relaxing Linearity 60
5.1.2 Relaxing Additivity 61
5.1.3 Model Overfitting 62
5.2 Bayesian Kernel Machine Regression (BKMR) 63
5.2.1 Introduction 63
5.2.2 Estimation 64
5.2.3 Variable Selection Procedures 64
5.2.4 Exposure-Outcome Function Characterization 67
5.2.5 Notes on Software Implementation 71
5.2.6 Recent Extensions of the BKMR Framework 72
5.2.7 BKMR: Concluding Remarks 73
5.3 Generalized Additive Models (GAMs) and Their Extensions 74
5.3.1 Introduction 74
5.3.2 GAM with Variable Selection 75
5.3.3 Bayesian Approaches for Penalized GAM 76
5.3.4 GAM: Concluding Remarks 77
5.4 Machine Learning for Environmental Mixtures 77
5.4.1 General Overview of Machine Learning Approaches 78
5.4.2 Areas of Interest in the Analysis of Environmental Mixtures 79
5.4.3 Machine Learning: Concluding Remarks 80
References 81

6 Additional Topics and Final Remarks 89
6.1 Causal Effects of Environmental Mixtures 89
6.1.1 A Note on Confounding and Effect Modification 90

6.2 Mediation Analysis to Assess the Role of Environmental Mixtures Within the Exposome 91
6.3 Incorporating Binary and Zero-Inflated Exposures........ 92
6.4 General Overview of Recent Methodological Advancements 93
6.5 Final Remarks: Analyses Plans for Mixture Studies in Environmental Epidemiology 94
6.5.1 Conclusion 95
References 96

Acronyms

BKMR	Bayesian Kernel Machine Regression
CV	Cross Validation
DAG	Directed Acyclic Graphs
GAM	Generalized Additive Model
GLM	Generalized Linear Model
LOD	Limit of Detection
MCMC	Markov Chain Monte Carlo
ML	Machine Learning
MSE	Mean Squared Error
NHANES	National Health and Nutrition Examination Survey
NIEHS	National Institute of Environmental Health Sciences
OLS	Ordinary Least Squares
PCA	Principal Component Analysis
PIP	Posterior Inclusion Probability
SD	Standard Deviation
VIF	Variance Inflation Factor
WQS	Weighted Quantile Sum

Chapter 1
Environmental Mixtures

1.1 Environmental Mixtures Within the Exposome Framework

Environmental epidemiology is the study of how factors in the external environment, including physical, biological, and chemical stressors, affect human health [12]. Levels of exposure to harmful environmental toxicants such as air and water pollutants, metals, and chemical components have been consistently rising over the last decades, contributing to an increased worldwide burden of several health conditions [22, 27]. The mechanisms through which environmental exposures affect human physiology are complex and involve several molecular pathways such as epigenetics mechanisms, genome-environment interactions, endocrine disruption, and microbiome alterations [2, 8, 10, 36]. Moreover, additional challenges when studying the effects of these external stressors come from the fact that individuals are simultaneously exposed to countless of these environmental factors, which jointly operate as determinants of health. The concept of *exposome* has been recently introduced to describe this complex and diverse set of exposures, incorporating dietary constituents, environmental factors, lifestyle, social, and other ecological factors, to which humans are exposed throughout their lifetime [13, 34, 35]. Within this context, to enable targeted prevention and interventions, the study of environmental factors as determinants of health should attempt to integrate individual differences in exposure and response that arise from these complex and heterogeneous individual exposure profiles [3].

Chemical stressors such as environmental pollutants, metals, or persistent and nonpersistent chemicals represent a substantial and key component of the exposome [3, 34]. A group of more than one chemical is commonly referred to as a chemical *mixture* [6, 26, 32]. Throughout this book we will use the terminology *environmental mixtures* to broadly indicate groups of individual chemicals designated as a combined entity [29]. In practice, groupings of chemicals are often defined based on chemical families (e.g., pollutant mixtures, phthalate mixtures, metal mixtures)

A. Bellavia, *Statistical Methods for Environmental Mixtures*, Society, Environment and Statistics, https://doi.org/10.1007/978-3-031-78987-8_1

of different dimensions and characterization based on specific data settings and research questions of interest [6, 29]. Assessing the health effects of environmental exposures as mixtures is critical to fully understand the way external factors operate on human physiology and is necessary to provide a more robust and realistic scientific basis for policy regulations [6]. The relevance of environmental mixtures in risk assessment has been long acknowledged, and toxicological studies on environmental stressors have integrated the assessment of chemicals as combined mixtures for several decades [9, 17, 20, 25, 26, 30, 32].

1.2 Mixtures Assessment in Environmental Epidemiology

In contrast to toxicological research, environmental epidemiology studies evaluating the health effects of environmental exposures in the general population have relied on assessing individual chemicals for a much longer time. One of the main reasons for this delayed transition to a multi-chemical mindset was certainly related to the analytical challenges that assessing complex environmental mixtures in population-based studies implicates. Commentaries and research papers encouraging a transition from single-chemical to multi-chemical approaches in epidemiologic studies started appearing in the early 2010s [4, 5, 7, 16, 28] initiating an extensive assessment of the limitations of standard statistical methodologies and of alternative approaches that could address the complexities of environmental mixtures. Governmental agencies such as the National Institute of Environmental Health Sciences (NIEHS) in the United States (US) included the development of statistical methodologies for environmental mixtures as a research priority [7, 28], further motivating researchers in the field to focus their effort on the development of ad hoc statistical methodologies.

A first comprehensive comparison of existing and novel methodologies for assessing the health effects of environmental mixtures was conducted in 2015 in a NIEHS workshop where 30 different approaches were compared [33]. The main conclusion of this pivotal workshop was that none of the evaluated approaches outperformed all other methods. Rather, the complexity of environmental mixtures requires a *triangulation* approach where several methodologies should be considered, each providing specific advantages to address different perspectives of the health effects of a certain mixture. Ensuing efforts to compare and review statistical methods for environmental mixtures have largely confirmed this result, underlying how different complementing approaches are required to address the several different research questions that should be considered for a comprehensive assessment of mixture-health associations [1, 11, 14, 19, 31]. Within this context, the first key step is to detail these distinct research questions and understand the different angles that they provide to the assessment of environmental mixtures and their effects.

1.3 Questions of Interest in Mixtures Research

As an illustrative example, we consider a study where the goal is to evaluate the effects of parabens—endocrine-disrupting chemicals commonly used in the production of personal care products and cosmetics—on the risk of developing diabetes in a specific population. Let's assume that through urine sample analyses we were able to assess concentration levels of a mixture of three common paraben compounds (methylparaben, butylparaben, propylparaben). A comprehensive assessment of the paraben mixtures and its effects on the risk of diabetes should address the following points.

1. *Patterns of Exposures*
   With several factors at play, it is often of interest to understand whether specific components of a chemical mixture are clustered into smaller subgroups, based on similar characteristics, shared sources, or other features. For example, are individuals with high levels of methylparaben more likely to also have higher levels of exposure to the other two compounds? The study of patterns of exposures provides relevant insights that can be integrated in subsequent analysis, but also contains information that can already inform policies, regulations, and interventions. For example, patterns of exposures that reflect shared sources provide information on modifiable factors that could be targeted to reduce exposure levels in the population (e.g., the use of unsafe personal care products).
2. *Cumulative Mixture Effect*
   A major goal of population-based studies is to understand the effects of environmental exposures in the general population and to identify potential interventions and recommendations. For a given individual, the specific levels of exposures to environmental chemicals are usually determined by the different sources that the individual is exposed to (e.g., the use of unsafe products in the paraben example, or living in a polluted neighborhood). These modifiable sources would likely represent the target of potential interventions and recommendations aimed at reducing overall levels of exposures to harmful chemicals in the population. Within this context, a primary question of interest is often the study of the *cumulative effect* of the mixture. Using the paraben example, what is the effect of exposure to the mixture of interest on the risk of developing diabetes? This cumulative effect will be the result of the complex molecular mechanisms associated with one or more of the three paraben compounds, but disentangling these mechanisms is not strictly necessary to provide an assessment of the overall effects of multiple chemicals and the potential interventions targeting sources of mixtures exposures.
3. *Mixtures' Bad Actors*
   On the other side of the coin, understanding the specific role of each chemical within the mixture of interest provides complementary information that might be of interest in several settings. Let's assume that our previous point has identified the presence of a cumulative effect of parabens on the risk of diabetes. This information might be enough to provide general recommendations (e.g.,

avoid paraben-containing products), but regulatory agencies will likely require additional information. Should policies be implemented to reduce levels of all mixtures components or just one of them? Which specific chemical would provide the largest risk reduction if eliminated from the source? Should individuals pay attention to products containing specific chemicals or any paraben? These questions relate to the identification of the *bad actors* within the mixture. Of note, this is of relevance even in the presence of a null cumulative effect, which might be the result of forces operating in different directions. Certain mixtures might include chemicals that are expected to operate in same directions, but more complex settings might well include components with positive effects on the outcome together with components that have a negative effect.

4. *Non-linear and Non-additive Effects*
   The cumulative effect of the mixture, whether negative, null, or positive, is the product of the several biological mechanisms associated with each of its components. As the mixture dimensionality increases, these mechanisms will likely include complex settings that involve non-linear and non-additive effects within the several chemicals. Not only these specific mechanisms are of interest from a toxicological perspective, but they should also be integrated, if present, for an unbiased assessment of cumulative effects. Assessing the presence of non-linear effects is of particular importance to understand whether there are thresholds of exposures that can be considered safe or whether also low levels of exposures should be considered harmful [15].

1.4 Structure of the Book

Over the last decade, following the abovementioned NIEHS workshop and the kickoff of several initiatives, the field of environmental epidemiology has gradually operated this transition from a single-chemical to multi-chemical mindset. The several methodological advancements that have been presented provide a wide array of tools for assessing the health effects of environmental mixtures under the different perspective described in Sect. 1.3 [18, 21]. More recent benchmark studies that have further incorporated novel approaches and extensions of existing ones have confirmed the conclusion that no method outperforms the others and that the choice of what approach to use should be guided by key considerations on data structures and research questions of interest [18, 23, 24, 37, 38]. This book follows this principle. The methods discussed over the next few chapters should not be regarded as a gradual improvement from basic to advanced approaches but rather as distinct tools that can be used within the same dataset to provide a robust understanding of mixture-health effects under different angles.

The several statistical approaches that have been proposed for assessing mixture effects attempt to target one or more of the research questions described in Sect. 1.3. A first classification of these approaches is between methods that do or do not take into account the relationship between the mixture and the outcome of interest.

Chapter 2 will focus on the former, discussing approaches for preliminary analysis and mixture characterization such as the identification of exposure patterns.

Subsequent chapters will incorporate the outcome of interest and discuss methods for assessing mixture-health associations. The common goal of all approaches that integrate health outcomes is to reduce the complexity of the data to be able to assess mixture-outcome associations while losing as little information as possible. This is broadly accomplished in two ways: by summarizing the original exposures into fewer covariates and by operating variable selection. Approaches for *variable selection* based on regression modeling will be the focus of Chap. 3. Techniques that reduce the dimension of the mixture by generating new variables, mostly relying on *indexing* and *dimensionality reduction*, will instead be the focus of Chap. 4.

A final important classification is between those approaches that are based on regression modeling versus nonparametric approaches that relax regression assumption to incorporate the flexibility required in complex settings. While the focus of Chaps. 3 and 4 will mostly be on regression-based approaches, flexible methods for complex settings will be discussed in Chap. 5.

Finally, together with some final considerations, Chap. 6 will summarize the described approaches and discuss how these different perspectives should be taken into account when designing analytical plans for mixture-health studies under different data settings of varying complexity.

1.5 Illustrative Example and Software Material

For all major approaches discussed, we will accompany the introduction to the method with its application on an illustrative example. This is based on a publicly available simulated dataset that was developed for the 2015 NIEHS workshop [33].[1] The data includes a mixture of 14 continuous exposures, $(X_1 - X_{14})$, a continuous outcome Y, and 3 additional covariates $(Z_1 - Z_3)$. Chemical distributions and correlation structure of the 14 mixture components were generated based on a mixture of polychlorinated biphenyls, dioxins, and furans, from the National Health and Nutrition Examination Survey (NHANES). Two clusters of highly correlated covariates were present $(X_3 - X_4 - X_5$, and $X_{12} - X_{13})$, while low to moderate correlations were simulated between all other covariates. Z_1 and Z_2 were simulated based on poverty index and age, both assumed to be confounders of the association. Z_3 was simulated based on biological sex distribution, and assumed to be an effect modifier. The outcome was generated with the following functions for men $(Z_3 = 0)$ and women $(Z_3 = 1)$, respectively:

- $E[Y] = 3+0.05 \cdot X_4+0.1 \cdot X_6+0.1 \cdot X_{11}+0.5 \cdot X_{12}+0.1 \cdot X_{14}+0.01 \cdot Z_1+0.003 \cdot Z_2$, for $Z_3 = 0$

[1] Hereafter referred to as *NHANES dataset*.

- $E[Y] = 3 + 0.01 \cdot X_1 + 0.05 \cdot X_4 + 0.1 \cdot X_{11} + 0.1 \cdot X_{14} + 0.01 \cdot Z_1 + 0.003 \cdot Z_2 - 0.32 \cdot (Z_3 = 1)$ for $Z_3 = 1$

Thus, for $Z_3 = 0$, only X_4, X_6, X_{11}, X_{12} and X_{14} are positively associated with Y. When $Z_3 = 1$, only X_1, X_4, X_{11} and X_{14} are associated with Y. Interactions between chemicals were not considered.

Most of the approaches developed and extended for the analysis of environmental mixtures, including all methods discussed in details in this book, can be implemented in the R statistical software. Codes to replicate all analyses presented in the book for the illustrative example, together with the simulated dataset, are available on https://github.com/andreabellavia/statsmixtures. The web page also includes updated links to online documentation and tutorials for several additional approaches.

References

1. Lydiane Agier, Lützen Portengen, Marc Chadeau-Hyam, Xavier Basagaña, Lise Giorgis-Allemand, Valérie Siroux, Oliver Robinson, Jelle Vlaanderen, Juan R González, Mark J Nieuwenhuijsen, et al. A systematic comparison of linear regression–based statistical methods to assess exposome-health associations. *Environmental health perspectives*, 124(12):1848–1856, 2016.
2. Janelle S Ayres. The biology of physiological health. *Cell*, 181(2):250–269, 2020.
3. Andrea Baccarelli, Dana C Dolinoy, and Cheryl Lyn Walker. A precision environmental health approach to prevention of human disease. *Nature Communications*, 14(1):2449, 2023.
4. Cécile Billionnet, Duane Sherrill, Isabella Annesi-Maesano, et al. Estimating the health effects of exposure to multi-pollutant mixture. *Annals of epidemiology*, 22(2):126–141, 2012.
5. Joseph M Braun, Chris Gennings, Russ Hauser, and Thomas F Webster. What can epidemiological studies tell us about the impact of chemical mixtures on human health? *Environmental health perspectives*, 124(1):A6–A9, 2016.
6. Danielle J Carlin and Cynthia V Rider. Combined exposures and mixtures research: An enduring NIEHS priority. *Environmental Health Perspectives*, 132(7):075001, 2024.
7. Danielle J Carlin, Cynthia V Rider, Rick Woychik, and Linda S Birnbaum. Unraveling the health effects of environmental mixtures: an niehs priority, 2013.
8. Cristina Casals-Casas and Béatrice Desvergne. Endocrine disruptors: from endocrine to metabolic disruption. *Annual review of physiology*, 73(1):135–162, 2011.
9. Nina Cedergreen. Quantifying synergy: a systematic review of mixture toxicity studies within environmental toxicology. *PloS One*, 9(5):e96580, 2014.
10. Karen Chiu, Genoa Warner, Romana A Nowak, Jodi A Flaws, and Wenyan Mei. The impact of environmental chemicals on the gut microbiome. *Toxicological Sciences*, 176(2):253–284, 2020.
11. Yu-Han Chiu, Andrea Bellavia, Tamarra James-Todd, Katharine F Correia, Linda Valeri, Carmen Messerlian, Jennifer B Ford, Lidia Mínguez-Alarcón, Antonia M Calafat, Russ Hauser, et al. Evaluating effects of prenatal exposure to phthalate mixtures on birth weight: A comparison of three statistical approaches. *Environment international*, 113:231–239, 2018.
12. National Research Council, Division on Earth, Life Studies, Commission on Life Sciences, Board on Environmental Studies, and Committee on Environmental Epidemiology. Environmental epidemiology, volume 1: Public health and hazardous wastes. 1991.
13. Yuxia Cui, David M Balshaw, Richard K Kwok, Claudia L Thompson, Gwen W Collman, and Linda S Birnbaum. The exposome: embracing the complexity for discovery in environmental health. *Environmental health perspectives*, 124(8):A137–A140, 2016.

14. Angel D Davalos, Thomas J Luben, Amy H Herring, and Jason D Sacks. Current approaches used in epidemiologic studies to examine short-term multipollutant air pollution exposures. *Annals of epidemiology*, 27(2):145–153, 2017.
15. Qian Di, Yan Wang, Antonella Zanobetti, Yun Wang, Petros Koutrakis, Christine Choirat, Francesca Dominici, and Joel D Schwartz. Air pollution and mortality in the medicare population. *New England Journal of Medicine*, 376(26):2513–2522, 2017.
16. Francesca Dominici, Roger D Peng, Christopher D Barr, and Michelle L Bell. Protecting human health from air pollution: shifting from a single-pollutant to a multipollutant approach. *Epidemiology*, 21(2):187–194, 2010.
17. Chris Gennings, Walter H Carter, Julie A Campain, Dong-soon Bae, and Raymond SH Yang. Statistical analysis of interactive cytotoxicity in human epidermal keratinocytes following exposure to a mixture of four metals. *Journal of Agricultural, Biological, and Environmental Statistics*, 7:58–73, 2002.
18. Elizabeth A Gibson, Yanelli Nunez, Ahlam Abuawad, Ami R Zota, Stefano Renzetti, Katrina L Devick, Chris Gennings, Jeff Goldsmith, Brent A Coull, and Marianthi-Anna Kioumourtzoglou. An overview of methods to address distinct research questions on environmental mixtures: an application to persistent organic pollutants and leukocyte telomere length. *Environmental Health*, 18:1–16, 2019.
19. Ghassan B Hamra and Jessie P Buckley. Environmental exposure mixtures: questions and methods to address them. *Current epidemiology reports*, 5(2):160–165, 2018.
20. Virginia Stewart Houk and Michael D Waters. Genetic toxicology and risk assessment of complex environmental mixtures. *Drug and chemical toxicology*, 19(3):187–219, 1996.
21. Bonnie R Joubert, Marianthi-Anna Kioumourtzoglou, Toccara Chamberlain, Hua Yun Chen, Chris Gennings, Mary E Turyk, Marie Lynn Miranda, Thomas F Webster, Katherine B Ensor, David B Dunson, et al. Powering research through innovative methods for mixtures in epidemiology (prime) program: novel and expanded statistical methods. *International Journal of Environmental Research and Public Health*, 19(3):1378, 2022.
22. Philip J Landrigan, Richard Fuller, Nereus JR Acosta, Olusoji Adeyi, Robert Arnold, Abdoulaye Bibi Baldé, Roberto Bertollini, Stephan Bose-O'Reilly, Jo Ivey Boufford, Patrick N Breysse, et al. The lancet commission on pollution and health. *The lancet*, 391(10119):462–512, 2018.
23. Nina Lazarevic, Adrian G Barnett, Peter D Sly, and Luke D Knibbs. Statistical methodology in studies of prenatal exposure to mixtures of endocrine-disrupting chemicals: a review of existing approaches and new alternatives. *Environmental health perspectives*, 127(2):026001, 2019.
24. Léa Maitre, Jean-Baptiste Guimbaud, Charline Warembourg, Nuria Güil-Oumrait, Paula Marcela Petrone, Marc Chadeau-Hyam, Martine Vrijheid, Xavier Basagaña, Juan R Gonzalez, Exposome Data Challenge Participant Consortium, et al. State-of-the-art methods for exposure-health studies: results from the exposome data challenge event. *Environment international*, 168:107422, 2022.
25. Joe L Mauderly. Toxicological approaches to complex mixtures. *Environmental health perspectives*, 101(suppl 4):155–165, 1993.
26. Emily Monosson. Chemical mixtures: considering the evolution of toxicology and chemical assessment. *Environmental health perspectives*, 113(4):383–390, 2005.
27. Annette Prüss-Ustün, Emilie van Deventer, Pierpaolo Mudu, Diarmid Campbell-Lendrum, Carolyn Vickers, Ivan Ivanov, Francesco Forastiere, Sophie Gumy, Carlos Dora, Heather Adair-Rohani, et al. Environmental risks and non-communicable diseases. *Bmj*, 364, 2019.
28. Cynthia V Rider, Danielle J Carlin, Micheal J DeVito, Claudia L Thompson, and Nigel J Walker. Mixtures research at NIEHS: an evolving program. *Toxicology*, 313(2–3):94–102, 2013.
29. David A Savitz and Anne M Hattersley. Evaluating chemical mixtures in epidemiological studies to inform regulatory decisions. *Environmental health perspectives*, 131(4):045001, 2023.
30. David J Spurgeon, Oliver AH Jones, Jean-Lou CM Dorne, Claus Svendsen, Suresh Swain, and Stephen R Stürzenbaum. Systems toxicology approaches for understanding the joint effects of

environmental chemical mixtures. *Science of the total environment*, 408(18):3725–3734, 2010.
31. Massimo Stafoggia, Susanne Breitner, Regina Hampel, and Xavier Basagaña. Statistical approaches to address multi-pollutant mixtures and multiple exposures: the state of the science. *Current environmental health reports*, 4(4):481–490, 2017.
32. William A Suk, Kenneth Olden, and Raymond SH Yang. Chemical mixtures research: significance and future perspectives. *Environmental Health Perspectives*, 110(suppl 6):891–892, 2002.
33. Kyla W Taylor, Bonnie R Joubert, Joe M Braun, Caroline Dilworth, Chris Gennings, Russ Hauser, Jerry J Heindel, Cynthia V Rider, Thomas F Webster, and Danielle J Carlin. Statistical approaches for assessing health effects of environmental chemical mixtures in epidemiology: lessons from an innovative workshop. *Environmental health perspectives*, 124(12):A227–A229, 2016.
34. Roel Vermeulen, Emma L Schymanski, Albert-László Barabási, and Gary W Miller. The exposome and health: Where chemistry meets biology. *Science*, 367(6476):392–396, 2020.
35. Christopher Paul Wild. Complementing the genome with an "exposome": the outstanding challenge of environmental exposure measurement in molecular epidemiology. *Cancer Epidemiology Biomarkers & Prevention*, 14(8):1847–1850, 2005.
36. Haotian Wu, Christina M Eckhardt, and Andrea A Baccarelli. Molecular mechanisms of environmental exposures and human disease. *Nature reviews genetics*, 24(5):332–344, 2023.
37. Linling Yu, Wei Liu, Xing Wang, Zi Ye, Qiyou Tan, Weihong Qiu, Xiuquan Nie, Minjing Li, Bin Wang, and Weihong Chen. A review of practical statistical methods used in epidemiological studies to estimate the health effects of multi-pollutant mixture. *Environmental Pollution*, 306:119356, 2022.
38. Guiming Zhu, Yanchao Wen, Kexin Cao, Simin He, and Tong Wang. A review of common statistical methods for dealing with multiple pollutant mixtures and multiple exposures. *Frontiers in Public Health*, 12:1377685, 2024.

Chapter 2
Characterizing Environmental Mixtures

2.1 Overview of Unsupervised Analyses for Environmental Mixtures

The previous chapter introduced the complexity of environmental mixtures and the several research questions that should be taken into account for a comprehensive assessment of their distribution in the population of interest and their effects on human health. Sections 1.2 and 1.3, in particular, discussed how the statistical analysis of environmental mixtures should involve several analytical steps that integrate multiple approaches to target the complexity of the potential research questions of interest. The goal of this chapter is to discuss the first critical step of any analytical plan: the characterization of the environmental mixtures. To fully understand the effects of complex mixture exposures on human health, it is necessary to first investigate and describe the properties of each individual component. This is achieved through a phase of *preprocessing*, which is necessary to identify potential complexities of specific chemicals that need to be addressed before investigating the mixture as a whole. Next, switching the focus to the environmental mixture as a whole, a set of analytical tools should be considered to (i) identify the distributions of exposures as they appear together in the population and (ii) to explore whether specific patterns of exposure are observed in the data. Borrowing terminology from the field of computer science, we can refer to this set of analytical steps as *unsupervised analysis*, indicating the different analyses conducted on the mixtures before taking into account its relationship with a health outcome [7]. Unsupervised analysis allows addressing some key research questions in the context of environmental mixtures but also provides results that can be used to inform subsequent steps focusing on mixture-health associations (supervised analysis). As such, unsupervised analyses presented in this chapter are an essential analytical step for any setting of interest in environmental mixtures modeling, with higher importance as the complexity and dimensionality of the mixture increases.

A. Bellavia, *Statistical Methods for Environmental Mixtures*, Society, Environment and Statistics, https://doi.org/10.1007/978-3-031-78987-8_2

Ideally, a comprehensive set of unsupervised analyses should at least include the following three steps:

1. Data preprocessing
2. Correlation analysis
3. Exposure pattern identification

2.2 Data Preprocessing

Before getting into the analysis of the environmental mixture, it is important to carefully assess its various components independently. Environmental exposures such as chemicals or pollutants, but also indicators of greenness, noise, or temperature, share important properties of analytical consequences that should be thoroughly explored.[1]

Skewness and High Variance
Skewness is a measure of the asymmetry of a continuous distribution. Environmental exposures are generally nonnegative and heavily skewed on the right, often presenting a high chance of observing distribution outliers. Normality of the distributions is required by most regression models for continuous outcomes, but can also offer advantages in terms of results interpretation for continuous exposures [12]. Logarithmic transformations of mixture components, for example, can be used to make skewed variables look more normal, as presented in Fig. 2.1 for one of the exposures in the NHANES data.[2] Log-transforming the original covariates, however, might hinder results interpretation when these are included in regression models, especially when the natural logarithm is used. As such, these transformations should not be applied as a default option but need to be considered on a case-by-case setting [3]. Of practical note, it is important to check for the presence of zero values before operating log transformations of continuous covariates.

Standardization
Different components of the same environmental mixture will often have different scales and levels of variability. For example, when assessing urinary concentrations of phthalate metabolites in the general US population, it is common to observe substantial heterogeneity with respect to the distribution of the different chemicals, with some metabolite distributions ranging from ~30 to ~4000 ug/L (e.g., monoethyl

[1] Throughout this and the following chapters, we will assume that mixture components are represented by continuous exposures, which is the natural format of chemicals and pollutant concentrations in most cases. Some notes on the specific case of zero-inflated and binary exposures are provided in Sect. 6.3.

[2] Log transformations are used for all analyses presented in the book. For simplicity, we will use the actual variables name (e.g., X_1) to indicate the log-transformed covariate.

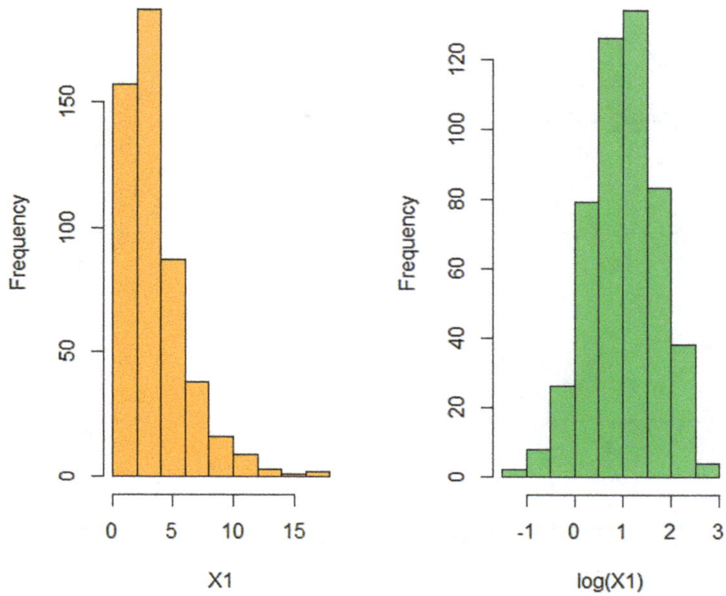

Fig. 2.1 Histogram of X_1 and $\log(X_1)$ in the NHANES dataset

phthalate—MEP) and other metabolites ranging from ∼1 to ∼20 ug/L (e.g., mono-(2-ethylhexyl) phthalate (MEHP)) [23]. These widely heterogeneous scales would not affect the interpretation of potential analysis on individual chemicals but do affect results interpretation when focusing on the mixture as a whole. Using this phthalate example, in a potential regression model that jointly includes both MEP and MEHP without transformations, the estimated coefficients expressing effects for a one-unit increase in each exposure might provide considerably larger results for MEHP. This, however, would be likely due to the fact that a one-unit increase in MEHP is a significant relative change (range: 1–20), while the same increase for MEP is not (range 30–4000). *Standardization* of mixture components is therefore required to fairly compare results from statistical models that incorporate them together. Specifically, for each component X, we transform individual values X_i by subtracting the average of X in the population and dividing by its SD: $\frac{X_i - mean(X)}{SD(X)}$. Figure 2.2 visually shows the effects of exposure standardization in a selected sample of covariates in the NHANES illustrative data. Of note, as for the case of log transformations, standardization will also require additional considerations when interpreting results from regression models or other supervised approaches.

Missing Values

A third key component of data processing is a thorough assessment of the distribution of missing data within the environmental mixture. This step is of particular relevance in our context of interest because the vast majority of statistical

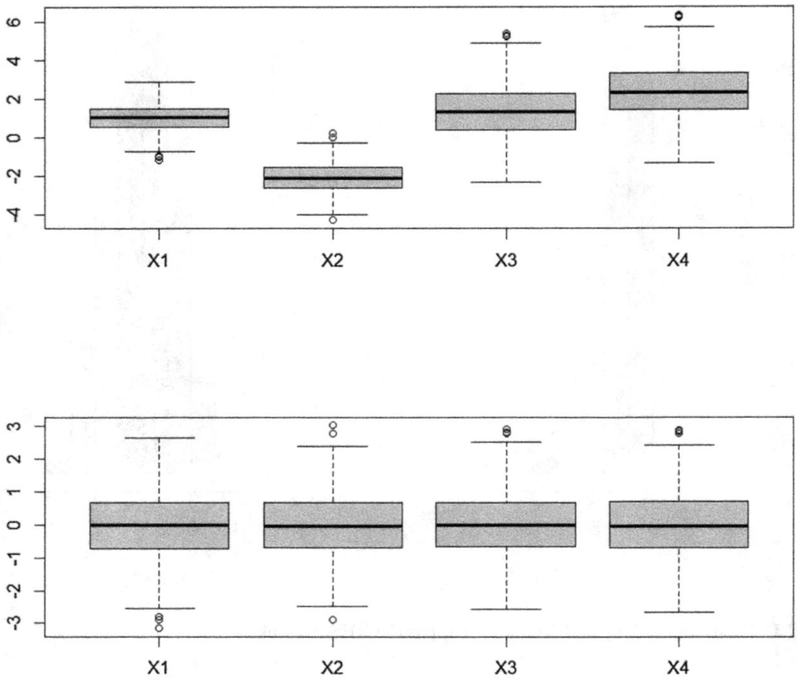

Fig. 2.2 Distribution of selected covariates in the NHANES dataset before (upper panel) and after (lower panel) standardization

approaches in the field will conduct a *complete-case* analysis restricting the data to the subsample of individuals with available information on all mixture components. For example, if we had a mixture of 10 exposures in a dataset of 1000 individuals, and 1 of these 10 components had 50% missing data, all analyses would be conducted on the restricted subsample of 500 individuals with complete data, with substantial loss of information. In this situation, researchers should select between one of these three options:

- Settle with the loss of power
- Remove the component with missing data from the mixture
- Impute missing values

Imputations techniques based on multiple imputations are only recommended if the proportion of missing data is not too high (10–15%) and will generally rely on the assumption that the missingness is at random [2].

Limits of Detection

Levels of concentrations of environmental chemicals are often assessed through sample analysis of human specimen. The laboratory technologies used to analyze the samples have general limitations in detecting low levels of concentrations [21].

For each substance of interest, the lowest concentration that can be discerned from zero is usually referred to as the *limit of detection* (LOD) [25]. Levels of concentrations under the LOD represent a very specific type of missing data where the reason for missingness is known. As such, classical imputation techniques that rely on assumptions of missingness at random are not a viable approach for this kind of situation. At the same time, there is often interest in understanding the effects of low levels of exposures, thus requiring the use of alternative imputation techniques. A common imputation approach for values under the LOD is to impute the constant value of $LOD/2$ or $LOD/\sqrt{2}$ [11]. This approach, however, is not exempt to some limitations. Especially in the presence of a high number of non-detected samples, imputing the same constant value to a high number of individuals will break the continuous nature of the covariate, with implications on their use in supervised approaches and interpretation [8]. Alternative procedures for imputing vales under the LOD in a more flexible way that also accounts for the multivariate nature of mixture exposures are available and should be considered in settings with complex patterns of missingness due to LOD [5, 6, 16, 17].

For the practical implementation of preprocessing steps for environmental mixtures, a recommended tool is the `rexposome` R package, described in detail in Hernandez-Ferrer et al. [9].

2.3 Correlation Analysis

Assessing the correlation structure between the mixture components is the first essential step when integrating environmental exposures together. Correlation analysis gives insights on the relationship between mixture components, allows a preliminary assessment of exposures patterns and clustering, and provides important information that can be integrated in subsequent modeling approaches.

For each pair of continuous covariates, a first visual assessment of their relationship can be observed using *scatterplots*. Figure 2.3, for example, shows a set of scatterplots for the NHANES data, where we observe some pairs of covariates highly associated within each other (e.g., X_3 and X_5), as well as pairs that seem to be completely independent (e.g., X_1 and X_5).

These figures provide some initial understanding of the likelihood of *co-exposure* to different mixture components. For example, individuals with high levels of concentrations of X_3 will almost certainly have higher levels of concentrations of X_5, possibly implying that the two environmental factors share one or more sources of exposures. Levels of concentrations of X_1 and X_5, on the other hand, seem to have no relationship in the data.

A *correlation coefficient* can be used to provide a quantitative assessment of these relationships. Two options can be considered. The Pearson correlation (r) measures the linear dependence between two variables, and it can only be used when both covariates are normally distributed:

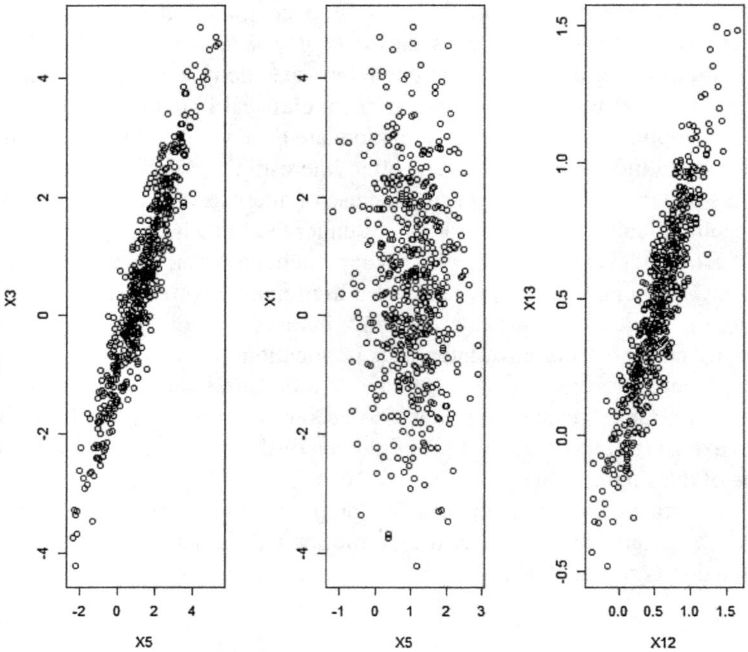

Fig. 2.3 Scatterplots of selected pairs of exposures in the NHANES dataset

$$r = \frac{\sum(X_1 - m_{X_1})(X_2 - m_{X_2})}{\sqrt{\sum(X_1 - m_{X_1})^2(X_2 - m_{X_2})^2}} \tag{2.1}$$

where m_{X_1} and m_{X_2} are the means of the two covariates X_1 and X_2.

The Spearman correlation (ρ) measures the correlation between the rank of the two covariates X_1 and X_2:

$$\rho = \frac{\sum(X_1' - m_{X_1'})(X_2' - m_{X_2'})}{\sqrt{\sum(X_1' - m_{X_1'})^2(X_2' - m_{X_2'})^2}} \tag{2.2}$$

where $m_{X_1'}$ and $m_{X_2'}$ are the means of the ranks of X_1 and X_2.

Spearman correlation is nonparametric and does not require assuming that the two evaluated covariates are normally distributed. As such, it allows detecting the direction of the monotonic relationship between the two covariates even if this relationship is not linear. For these reasons, Spearman correlation is usually preferred when evaluating environmental exposures. Both r and ρ are bounded between -1 and 1 (negative and positive correlation), with values of 0 indicating the absence of correlation. Tests for statistical significance of the correlation coefficient are available for both r and ρ, both comparing to the null hypothesis of no correlation.

When evaluating the correlation between several pairs of exposures, we can create a *correlation matrix*, displayed in Table 2.1 for the 14 exposures in the NHANES data. A better visualization of the correlation structure of the mixture can be obtained graphically by using a *correlation plot* (or correlogram; Fig. 2.4).

Table 2.1 Correlation matrix of mixture components in the NHANES dataset

	X_1	X_2	X_3	X_4	X_5	X_6	X_7	X_8	X_9	X_{10}	X_{11}	X_{12}	X_{13}	X_{14}
X_1	1.00	0.30	−0.04	−0.03	−0.03	0.04	0.16	−0.05	0.15	−0.10	−0.11	0.35	0.34	0.01
X_2	0.30	1.00	0.05	0.06	0.08	0.07	0.18	0.03	0.14	−0.02	−0.03	0.39	0.38	0.05
X_3	−0.04	0.05	1.00	0.99	0.93	0.60	0.28	0.74	0.17	0.40	0.56	−0.11	−0.14	0.70
X_4	−0.03	0.06	0.99	1.00	0.94	0.61	0.29	0.74	0.18	0.41	0.57	−0.09	−0.13	0.71
X_5	−0.03	0.08	0.93	0.94	1.00	0.59	0.29	0.72	0.17	0.42	0.56	−0.10	−0.14	0.69
X_6	0.04	0.07	0.60	0.61	0.59	1.00	0.46	0.64	0.38	0.45	0.54	0.06	0.03	0.62
X_7	0.16	0.18	0.28	0.29	0.29	0.46	1.00	0.39	0.70	0.36	0.41	0.46	0.48	0.41
X_8	−0.05	0.03	0.74	0.74	0.72	0.64	0.39	1.00	0.37	0.55	0.64	0.01	−0.03	0.74
X_9	0.15	0.14	0.17	0.18	0.17	0.38	0.70	0.37	1.00	0.32	0.36	0.50	0.50	0.40
X_{10}	−0.10	−0.02	0.40	0.41	0.42	0.45	0.36	0.55	0.32	1.00	0.77	0.00	−0.05	0.42
X_{11}	−0.11	−0.03	0.56	0.57	0.56	0.54	0.41	0.64	0.36	0.77	1.00	−0.01	−0.07	0.54
X_{12}	0.35	0.39	−0.11	−0.09	−0.10	0.06	0.46	0.01	0.50	0.00	−0.01	1.00	0.90	0.11
X_{13}	0.34	0.38	−0.14	−0.13	−0.14	0.03	0.48	−0.03	0.50	−0.05	−0.07	0.90	1.00	0.07
X_{14}	0.01	0.05	0.70	0.71	0.69	0.62	0.41	0.74	0.40	0.42	0.54	0.11	0.07	1.00

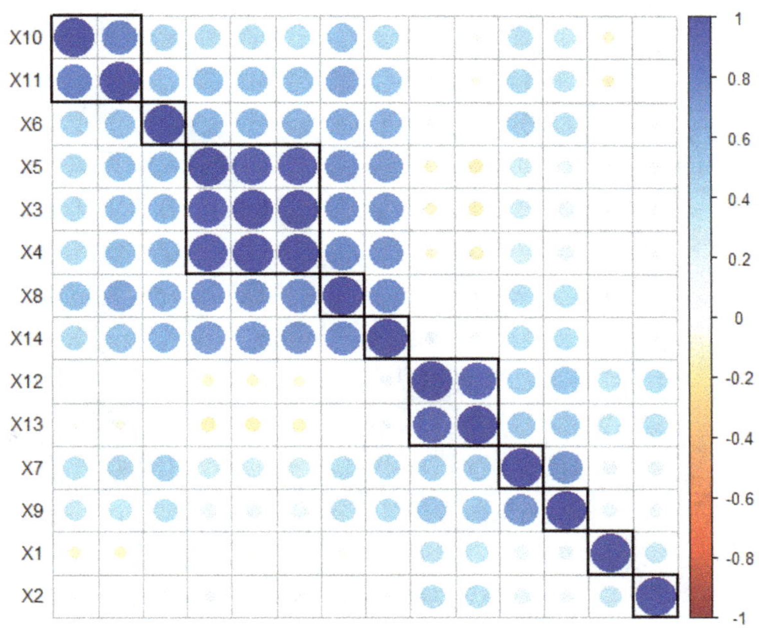

Fig. 2.4 Correlation plot of mixture components in the NHANES dataset

The correlation plot provides several important preliminary insights on the pattern of exposures to the mixture. Two clusters of highly correlated factors are identified: $X_3 - X_4 - X_5$; and $X_{12} - X_{13}$. Members of the first cluster also have moderate correlation levels with several other covariates (X_6, X_8, X_{10}, X_{11},X_{14}), while the second cluster is more isolated and only presents some additional levels of moderate correlations with X_7 and X_9. Finally, X_1 and X_2 do not display relevant levels of correlation with any other mixture components.

2.3.1 Correlation Network Analysis

Network analysis is a flexible and powerful visualization tool routinely used in different fields [10, 15]. A network is a complex structure of variables, called *nodes*, and of relationships (formally called *edges*) between these nodes. Correlation networks define such relationships on the basis of the quantitative correlations of the nodes, and are increasingly being used in biology to analyze high-dimensional datasets [24]. Weighted correlation networks, in particular, preserve the continuous nature of the underlying correlation information without dichotomizing information and can provide a better depiction of the correlation structure underlying the mixture as compared to a correlation plot, especially in the presence of high-dimensional mixtures. The correlation network of the 14 NHANES exposures is presented in Fig. 2.5.

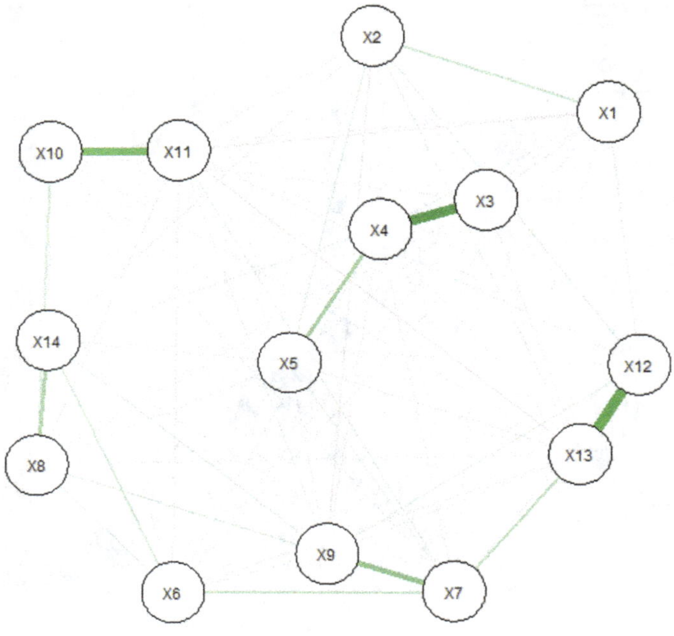

Fig. 2.5 Weighted correlation network of mixture components in the NHANES dataset

2.4 Principal Component Analysis: (PCA)

Principal component analysis (PCA) is a popular technique of exploratory data analysis for dimensionality reduction. The general goal of PCA is to reduce the original set of covariates into a smaller set of *principal components* that still contains most of the original information. This information is defined in terms of variability of a high-dimensional dataset that the smaller set of components should attempt to retrieve.

2.4.1 Principal Components Derivation

To understand the principles of PCA, it is useful to think of it in geometrical terms. Specifically, a principal component can be thought of as the direction in the covariate space where there is the most variance and the data is most spread out. Figure 2.6 provides a graphical overview of the data points in a simple setting of three mixture components (the maximum number the human mind can visualize geometrically). The way PCA derives a first principal component to describe the mixture is by identifying the straight line that best spreads the data out when it is projected along it, thus explaining the most substantial variance in the data.

In mathematical terms, this first component t_1 is calculated as a linear combination of the p original predictors $T = XW_p$, where W_p are weights that

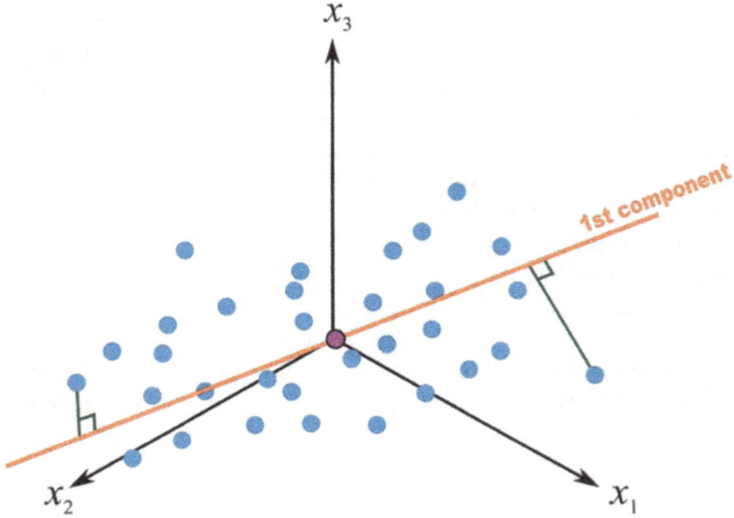

Fig. 2.6 First principal component in a three-covariate setting. Reproduced with permission from https://learnche.org/pid, Chap. 6.5

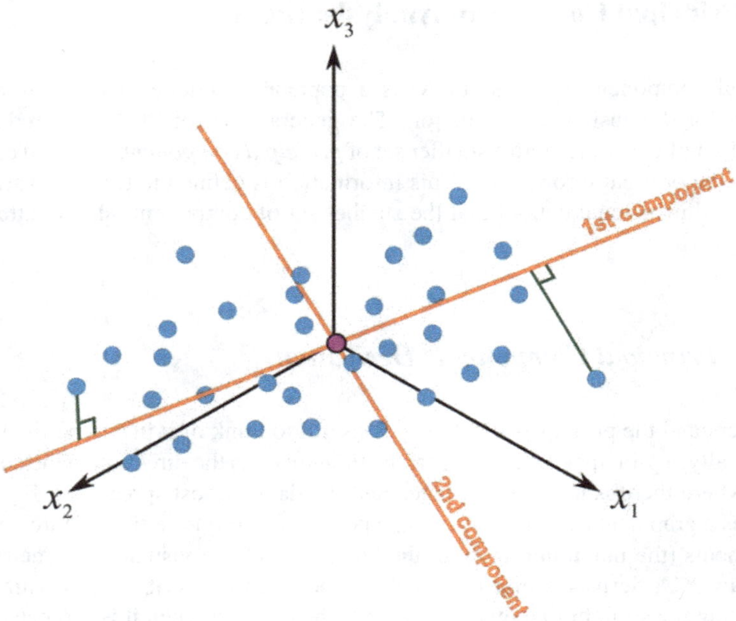

Fig. 2.7 Second principal component in a three-covariate setting. Reproduced with permission from https://learnche.org/pid, Chap. 6.5

would maximize the overall explained variability.[3] Once a first component has been retrieved, the PCA algorithm proceeds by calculating a second component that would maximize the residual variance. Of interest in our context, the procedure adds a constraint of *orthogonality* to this second component, that is, this second component will be uncorrelated to the first one, as presented in Fig. 2.7.

The algorithm then proceeds until a full set of p components that explain all the variability of the original p covariates are derived. In summary, PCA is a set of linear transformations that fits the matrix of exposures into a new coordinate system so that the most variance is explained by the first coordinate, and each subsequent coordinate is orthogonal to the previous ones and has a lesser variance. In practice, we are transforming a set of p correlated variables into a set of p uncorrelated principal components. PCA is sensitive to unscaled covariates, so it is usually recommended to standardize the matrix of exposures before fitting the model. PCA is available in several R packages including the aforementioned `rexposome` [9].

[3] Specifically, these weights are the *eigenvectors* of the correlation matrix of the original exposures. Understanding the complex mathematical concept of eigenvectors is not necessary to appreciate the practical relevance of PCA and will not be discussed further.

2.4.2 Choosing the Number of Components

One of the most appealing features of PCA is that, while it is possible to calculate p components from a set of p covariates, we usually need a smaller number to successfully describe most of the variance of the original matrix of exposures. In practical terms, not only we are reshaping the original set of exposures into uncorrelated principal components, but we might also be able to reduce the dimension of the original matrix into a smaller number of variables that can describe our mixture with limited loss of information.

To this extent, it is important to carefully consider how to select the number of components that should be retrieved. The following criteria are commonly considered:

- Selecting components that cumulatively explain at least 70–80% of the original data variability
- Selecting components whose individual measure of variance is larger than 1
- Selecting components based on the inflation point in the graphical display of the components variance (*scree plot*)

Before discussing these tools in the illustrative NHANES example, it is useful to stress that this choice will remain subjective. There might be settings where all criteria lead to the same evident conclusion as well as settings where it is not straightforward to identify a clear number of components that meaningfully describe the original data.

Table 2.2 reports results from fitting a PCA on the 14 NHANES exposures, including the proportion of mixture variance explained by each specific component and the cumulative variance explained. The scree plot is instead presented

Table 2.2 PCA: proportion of explained variance for all extracted principal components (PC) in the NHANES dataset

	Proportion of variance	Cumulative proportion
PC1	0.43320	0.43320
PC2	0.21928	0.65248
PC3	0.08971	0.74219
PC4	0.05758	0.79977
PC5	0.05029	0.85006
PC6	0.03738	0.88744
PC7	0.02913	0.91657
PC8	0.02594	0.94251
PC9	0.01710	0.95961
PC10	0.01515	0.97476
PC11	0.01356	0.98832
PC12	0.00632	0.99464
PC13	0.00466	0.99930
PC14	0.00070	1.00000

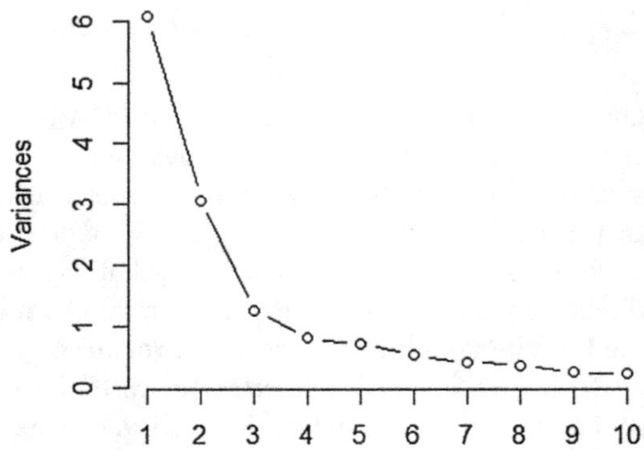

Fig. 2.8 Scree plot after fitting principal component analysis in the NHANES dataset

in Fig. 2.8. In this example, all three criteria seem to indicate that 3 principal components might be enough to comprehensively describe the original set of 14 exposures.

2.4.3 *Making Sense of Component Interpretation*

Broadly speaking, a PCA is composed of three analytical steps. The first step—deriving the components—despite the non-straightforward geometrical explanation of the procedure, can be easily conducted within a couple of lines of coding. The second step is the selection of how many components to retrieve, which requires some level of subjectivity guided by some quantitative criteria. The final major step, mostly subjective, requires interpreting the extracted principal components. Pivotal information to such end is provided by the *loading factors*, representing the correlation coefficients between the extracted components and the original covariates. These measures reflect how much of the original variance of each covariate is explained by each component. For a clear interpretation of loading factors, it is usually recommended to operate a technical transformation to the components called *axis rotation*. Several approaches for rotation are available and integrated and fully documented in the several R packages available to conduct PCA. Loading factors for the rotated versions of the three selected components in the NHANES dataset are presented in Table 2.3.

The three components seem to confirm the preliminary findings from the correlation analysis. We observe X_1, X_2 having higher loading on PC3, X_7, X_9, X_{12}, X_{13} loading on PC2, and all other exposures loading on PC1. Nevertheless, we do not observe a clear discrimination that would allow a meaningful labeling of the three components. This is not a problem but rather a conclusion that PCA is providing in terms of exposure patterns. Specifically, the first set of unsupervised analyses in the NHANES dataset indicates that the environmental mixture presents a complex correlation structure with no obvious patterns of exposures and clear discrimination

Table 2.3 PCA loading factors, presenting the correlation between the three selected principal components (PC) and the original covariates

	PC1	PC2	PC3
X_1	0.089	0.162	0.428
X_2	0.163	0.123	0.506
X_3	0.452	−0.102	0.081
X_4	0.455	−0.098	0.087
X_5	0.450	−0.098	0.093
X_6	0.275	0.105	−0.115
X_7	0.071	0.435	−0.152
X_8	0.332	0.062	−0.131
X_9	0.004	0.473	−0.198
X_{10}	0.097	0.178	−0.446
X_{11}	0.182	0.134	−0.382
X_{12}	−0.046	0.466	0.227
X_{13}	−0.074	0.473	0.218
X_{14}	0.332	0.099	−0.039

of the mixture components into distinct groups. In those settings where a clear interpretation was available, PCA results could instead be fed into several of the supervised approaches we will discuss over the next chapters.[4]

2.4.4 PCA: Concluding Remarks

PCA is a key component of the preliminary unsupervised assessment of the mixture. In addition to providing relevant information to subsequent analysis, there are several settings where PCA is used as a stand-alone approach to address questions of exposure patterns (see, e.g., [20] and [22]). Identifying exposure patterns has relevant implications from an epidemiologic and public health perspective. For example, identified patterns might suggest the presence of specific sources of exposures in the population of interest that could be the target of public health interventions and policy recommendations. As already mentioned, using PCA results into subsequent supervised analysis requires a meaningful and clear interpretation of the extracted components. For a practical illustration of component interpretation, see, for example, Minguez-Alarcon et al. [19], applying PCA on a mixture of endocrine-disrupting chemicals and identifying two components clearly summarizing the variability of di(2-ethylhexyl)phthalate (DEHP) vs non-DEHP metabolites, labeled as such for the subsequent analyses.

[4] Integrating PCA results into a regression model will be discussed in Sect. 4.2. PCA results can also be used to inform approaches that allow exposure groupings such as grouped LASSO (Sect. 3.3.5) and hierarchical BKMR (Sect. 5.2.3).

To strengthen the interpretation of the identified exposure patterns, additional unsupervised approaches can be incorporated. *Cluster analysis*, for example, can be used to group individuals, rather than covariates, based on similar levels of mixture of exposures [14]. Kalloo et al. [13] provide an excellent example of thorough unsupervised analysis in the context of environmental mixtures, integrating PCA and clustering with correlation analysis to identify patterns of environmental chemicals in a population of pregnant women.

A recent publication has discussed an alternative unsupervised approach for dimensionality reduction, namely, *principal component pursuit* (PCP), as a potential methodology for exposure pattern discoveries in the context of environmental mixtures [4]. This approach provides a flexible framework of high potential that has shown a substantial improvement over PCA based on preliminary simulations, especially in the presence of several non-detected values. To this date, applications of the approach are still limited [1, 26], and external validations and applications in different settings are required for a comprehensive appreciation of its advantages and limitations. Finally, for an overview of alternative approaches for dimensionality reduction that might represent useful tools to estimate exposure patterns and groupings between mixture components, the reader can refer to the recent review of Liu et al. [18].

References

1. Jaime Benavides, Sabah Usmani, Vijay Kumar, and Marianthi-Anna Kioumourtzoglou. Development of a community severance index for urban areas in the united states: A case study in new york city. *Environment international*, 185:108526, 2024.
2. James R Carpenter, Jonathan W Bartlett, Tim P Morris, Angela M Wood, Matteo Quartagno, and Michael G Kenward. *Multiple imputation and its application*. John Wiley & Sons, 2023.
3. Giehae Choi, Jessie P Buckley, Jordan R Kuiper, and Alexander P Keil. Log-transformation of independent variables: must we? *Epidemiology*, 33(6):843–853, 2022.
4. Elizabeth A Gibson, Junhui Zhang, Jingkai Yan, Lawrence Chillrud, Jaime Benavides, Yanelli Nunez, Julie B Herbstman, Jeff Goldsmith, John Wright, and Marianthi-Anna Kioumourtzoglou. Principal component pursuit for pattern identification in environmental mixtures. *Environmental Health Perspectives*, 130(11):117008, 2022.
5. Paul M Hargarten and David C Wheeler. Accounting for the uncertainty due to chemicals below the detection limit in mixture analysis. *Environmental research*, 186:109466, 2020.
6. Paul M Hargarten and David C Wheeler. miwqs: Multiple imputation using weighted quantile sum regression. *R J.*, 12(2):226, 2020.
7. Trevor Hastie, Robert Tibshirani, Jerome Friedman, Trevor Hastie, Robert Tibshirani, and Jerome Friedman. Unsupervised learning. *The elements of statistical learning: Data mining, inference, and prediction*, pages 485–585, 2009.
8. Dennis Helsel. Much ado about next to nothing: incorporating nondetects in science. *Annals of occupational hygiene*, 54(3):257–262, 2010.
9. Carles Hernandez-Ferrer, Gregory A Wellenius, Ibon Tamayo, Xavier Basagaña, Jordi Sunyer, Martine Vrijheid, and Juan R Gonzalez. Comprehensive study of the exposome and omic data using rexposome bioconductor packages. *Bioinformatics*, 35(24):5344–5345, 2019.
10. David Hevey. Network analysis: a brief overview and tutorial. *Health Psychology and Behavioral Medicine*, 6(1):301–328, 2018.

11. Richard W Hornung and Laurence D Reed. Estimation of average concentration in the presence of nondetectable values. *Applied Occupational and Environmental Hygiene*, 5(1):46–51, 1990.
12. Janice MY Hu, Liheng Harry Zhuang, Brendan A Bernardo, and Lawrence C McCandless. Statistical challenges in the analysis of biomarkers of environmental chemical exposures for perinatal epidemiology. *Current epidemiology reports*, 5:284–292, 2018.
13. Geetika Kalloo, Gregory A Wellenius, Lawrence McCandless, Antonia M Calafat, Andreas Sjodin, Margaret Karagas, Aimin Chen, Kimberly Yolton, Bruce P Lanphear, and Joseph M Braun. Profiles and predictors of environmental chemical mixture exposure among pregnant women: the health outcomes and measures of the environment study. *Environmental science & technology*, 52(17):10104–10113, 2018.
14. Leonard Kaufman and Peter J Rousseeuw. *Finding groups in data: an introduction to cluster analysis*. John Wiley & Sons, 2009.
15. Peter Langfelder and Steve Horvath. Wgcna: an r package for weighted correlation network analysis. *BMC bioinformatics*, 9(1):1–13, 2008.
16. Nathanael Lapidus, Sylvie Chevret, and Matthieu Resche-Rigon. Assessing assay agreement estimation for multiple left-censored data: a multiple imputation approach. *Statistics in Medicine*, 33(30):5298–5309, 2014.
17. Myeonggyun Lee, Abhisek Saha, Rajeshwari Sundaram, Paul S Albert, and Shanshan Zhao. Accommodating detection limits of multiple exposures in environmental mixture analyses: an overview of statistical approaches. *Environmental Health*, 23(1):48, 2024.
18. Shelley H Liu, Yitong Chen, Jordan R Kuiper, Emily Ho, Jessie P Buckley, and Leah Feuerstahler. Applying latent variable models to estimate cumulative exposure burden to chemical mixtures and identify latent exposure subgroups: A critical review and future directions. *Statistics in Biosciences*, pages 1–21, 2024.
19. Lidia Mínguez-Alarcón, Carmen Messerlian, Andrea Bellavia, Audrey J Gaskins, Yu-Han Chiu, Jennifer B Ford, Alexandra R Azevedo, John C Petrozza, Antonia M Calafat, Russ Hauser, et al. Urinary concentrations of bisphenol a, parabens and phthalate metabolite mixtures in relation to reproductive success among women undergoing in vitro fertilization. *Environment international*, 126:355–362, 2019.
20. Gila Neta, Lynn R Goldman, Dana Barr, Andreas Sjodin, Benjamin J Apelberg, Frank R Witter, and Rolf U Halden. Distribution and determinants of pesticide mixtures in cord serum using principal component analysis. *Environmental science & technology*, 44(14):5641–5648, 2010.
21. Eduard Rogatsky and Daniel Stein. Evaluation of matrix effect and chromatography efficiency: new parameters for validation of method development. *Journal of the American Society for Mass Spectrometry*, 16(11):1757–1759, 2005.
22. Astrid Schilmann, Marina Lacasaña, Julia Blanco-Muñoz, Clemente Aguilar-Garduño, Aarón Salinas-Rodríguez, Mario Flores-Aldana, and Mariano E Cebrián. Identifying pesticide use patterns among flower growers to assess occupational exposure to mixtures. *Occupational and environmental medicine*, 67(5):323–329, 2010.
23. Manori J Silva, Dana B Barr, John A Reidy, Nicole A Malek, Carolyn C Hodge, Samuel P Caudill, John W Brock, Larry L Needham, and Antonia M Calafat. Urinary levels of seven phthalate metabolites in the US population from the national health and nutrition examination survey (nhanes) 1999–2000. *Environmental health perspectives*, 112(3):331–338, 2004.
24. Dirk Steinhauser, Leonard Krall, Carsten Müssig, Dirk Büssis, and Björn Usadel. Correlation networks. *Analysis of biological networks*, 305:333, 2008.
25. Paul A. Succop, Scott Clark, Mei Chen, and Warren Galke. Imputation of data values that are less than a detection limit. *Journal of Occupational and Environmental Hygiene*, 1:436–441, 2004.
26. Haotian Wu, Vrinda Kalia, Katherine E Manz, Lawrence Chillrud, Nathalie Hoffmann Dishon, Gabriela L Jackson, Christian K Dye, Raoul Orvieto, Adva Aizer, Hagai Levine, et al. Exposome profiling of environmental pollutants in seminal plasma and novel associations with semen parameters. *Environmental Science & Technology*, 2024.

Chapter 3
Regression-Based Approaches for Mixture-Health Associations

3.1 Overview of Regression Modeling in Environmental Mixtures Research

The characterization of an environmental mixture through correlation analysis and exposure pattern discovery, described in the previous chapter, is often the first of several analytical steps. In the context of environmental epidemiology, researchers are generally interested to further investigate the extent to which exposure to these environmental mixtures is harmful to human health. Epidemiologists are trained to address questions of exposure-health associations using regression-based techniques such as generalized linear models (GLM), for binary and continuous outcomes, or parametric and semi-parametric regression techniques for time-to-event outcomes [15, 18]. Within this context, it was natural for earlier attempts in studying the health effects of environmental exposures as multifactorial mixtures to exploit the use of regression modeling. Over the last decades, several existing regression-based approaches have been investigated as potential tools for assessing mixture-health associations. The first section of this chapter presents the use of classical regression techniques (e.g., GLM) for modeling the association between an environmental mixture and a health outcome, and describes the challenges and limitations of these classical approaches in this context. The second section will then introduce penalized regression as an alternative regression framework that addresses some of the common shortcomings of GLM in mixture modeling. Finally, the last section will provide some general considerations on the research questions that regression modeling leaves unsettled and that have motivated researchers to develop ad hoc statistical approaches for environmental mixtures, which will be the focus of the following chapters.

A. Bellavia, *Statistical Methods for Environmental Mixtures*, Society, Environment and Statistics, https://doi.org/10.1007/978-3-031-78987-8_3

3.2 Classical Regression Approaches and Their Limitations

3.2.1 Environmental-Wide Association Studies

A simple way to assess the association between a set of p environmental exposures $(X_1 - X_p)$ and a given outcome Y is to build p different regression models, one for each mixture component, one at a time. Any classical regression model used in epidemiology can be chosen depending on the nature of the health outcome of interest (e.g., GLM, Cox regression). This *single-chemical* or *single-pollutant* approach has been the default analytical tool in environmental epidemiology for several decades [4, 8, 17]. Because of its similarity with genome-wide associations studies (GWAS), another common way of describing this methodology is as environmental-wide association studies [13, 23]. Each individual model can be further adjusted for potential confounders (C) of each exposure-outcome association. For example, with a continuous outcome Y, we could fit a set of linear regression models such as

$$Y_i = \beta_0 + \beta_1 \cdot X_{1i} + \beta \cdot C + \epsilon_i \tag{3.1}$$

where β_1 represents the estimated effect on the outcome associated with a one-unit increase in the exposure.

Assessing several regression models will increase the risk of false-positive findings. As in the case of GWAS, this issue is commonly addressed by adjusting for *multiple comparisons*, using common techniques such as Bonferroni adjustment and False Discovery Rate [13].

Single-chemical regressions implicitly make an important assumption that severely hampers their interpretation and applicability in population-based studies. Specifically, when assessing the association between one mixture component and the outcome, we are assuming that none of the other mixture components act as confounders of this exposure-outcome association. This can be depicted with the directed acyclic graph (DAG)[1] presented in Fig. 3.1.

3.2.2 Co-confounding Between Mixture Components

The confounding assumption made by single-chemical studies is seldom realistic. For example, high levels of correlation between mixture components (e.g., X_3, X_4, X_5 in the NHANES illustrative data) often indicate that these factors share one or more sources of exposures. Using the example of these three highly correlated covariates in the illustrative data, the real DAG used for simulating the data is presented in Fig. 3.2. where U is the source of exposure to the three factors

[1] DAGs are a useful tool in causal inference to depict the causal relationship between variables of interest. A gentle introduction to DAG can be found in Digitale et al. [7].

Fig. 3.1 Implicit causal assumptions of single-chemical regression models

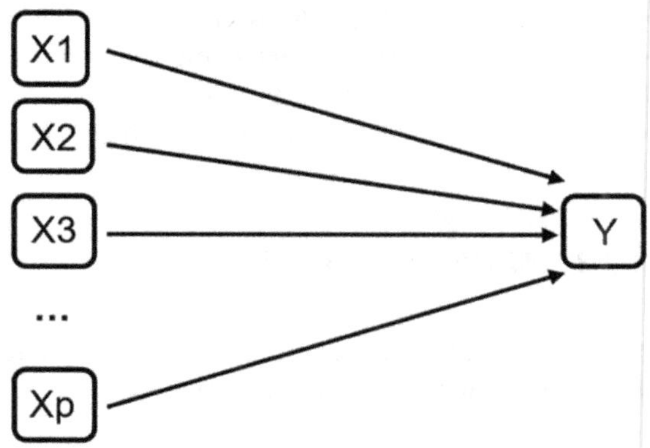

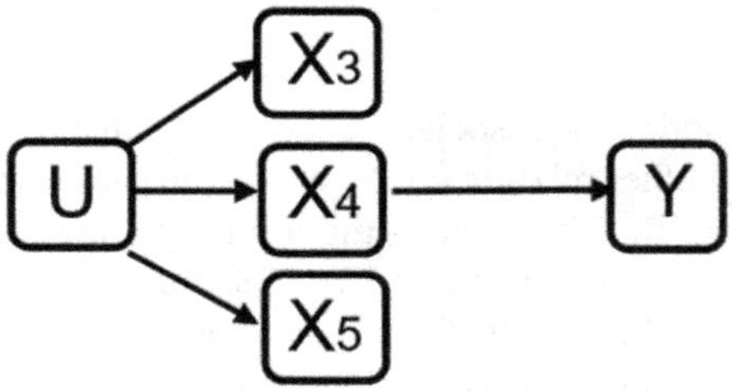

Fig. 3.2 DAG to describe the real causal relationship between X_3,X_4, X_5 and the outcome Y in the NHANES dataset. The three chemicals are highly correlated as they share a common source U. Out of the three, only X_4 has a causal effect on the outcome

Table 3.1 Results from individual regression models of three selected mixture components in the NHANES dataset

	Estimate	p-value
X_3	0.078	0.007
X_4	0.089	0.003
X_5	0.068	0.005

(e.g., a plastic container with three chemicals; living in a neighborhood with high levels of three pollutants).

Table 3.1, which reports results from individual regression models for these three predictors in the NHANES dataset, fails to capture that only one of the three exposures (X_4) is truly associated with the outcome and instead provides evidence of a potential association between each of the three factors and the outcome. The reason for this discrepancy is the fact that individual regression models are subject to confounding bias. For example, to assess the effect of X_5 on Y, we should adjust for X_4, which is both associated with the outcome and with X_5 (through the common source U).[2] In a real setting, where we do not know a priori which (if any) of

[2] For the reader familiar with causal inference terminology, the common source represents a *backdoor pathway* that should be blocked by adjusting for X_4.

the three exposures is really associated with the outcome, we should adjust each individual model for all other components of the mixture. This concept of *co-confounding* between mixture components is critical for a thorough assessment of who the real contributors to the mixture-health effect are.

3.2.3 Multiple Regression

The most intuitive way to account for this co-confounding is to *mutually adjust* for all exposures in the same regression model:

$$Y_i = \beta_0 + \sum_{j=1}^{p} \beta_j \cdot X_{ji} + \beta \cdot C + \epsilon_i \tag{3.2}$$

In this regression model, the association between each exposure and the outcome will be adjusted for all other mixture components, thus addressing the potential bias due to co-confounding. Results from fitting a multiple regression model mutually adjusting for the 14 exposures in the NHANES illustrative data are presented in Table 3.2, also including full results from individual models for comparison.

Results from the multiple regression are not consistent with those obtained from independent regression models, especially for those exposures that showed high levels of correlations. For example, just focusing on the nominal values of the estimates within the highly correlated group discussed before, X_4 is now (correctly) identified as being positively associated with Y. This improvement, however, often

Table 3.2 Multiple and single regression results in the NHANES dataset

	Estimate—multiple	p-value—multiple	Estimate—single	p-value—single
X_1	0.058	0.080	0.106	0.001
X_2	0.018	0.554	0.073	0.012
X_3	−0.030	0.774	0.078	0.007
X_4	0.053	0.644	0.089	0.003
X_5	0.004	0.923	0.068	0.005
X_6	0.060	0.047	0.120	<0.001
X_7	−0.031	0.620	0.153	<0.001
X_8	0.017	0.679	0.137	<0.001
X_9	0.025	0.673	0.160	<0.001
X_{10}	0.052	0.260	0.125	<0.001
X_{11}	0.049	0.341	0.149	<0.001
X_{12}	0.222	0.138	0.294	<0.001
X_{13}	−0.083	0.586	0.238	<0.001
X_{14}	0.054	0.293	0.185	<0.001

comes with new problems. In this data, for example, we are now observing some negative estimates, especially for covariates within correlated clusters (e.g., X_3 and X_{13}). We know that this is a wrong conclusion (all exposures have either null or positive effects), thanks to the simulated nature of the data, but in real settings we would still remain mostly clueless with respect to what the real contributors to the mixture-health effect, if any, really are.

3.2.4 Multicollinearity

Including highly correlated covariates in the same regression model increases the risk of *multicollinearity* (or simply *collinearity*). More specifically, a high correlation between two predictors simultaneously included in a regression model will decrease the precision of their estimates and increase their standard errors. Collinearity is due to the fact that when the correlation between two covariates (say X_1 and X_2) is very high, then one is a pretty accurate linear predictor of the other. A common consequence is that, if the two predictors X_1 and X_2 were really associated with the outcome (e.g., $\beta = 0.25$ for both), the actual estimates of their effect from multiple regression at varying levels of correlation between the two predictors $\rho(X_1, X_2)$ would likely behave as presented in Fig. 3.3.

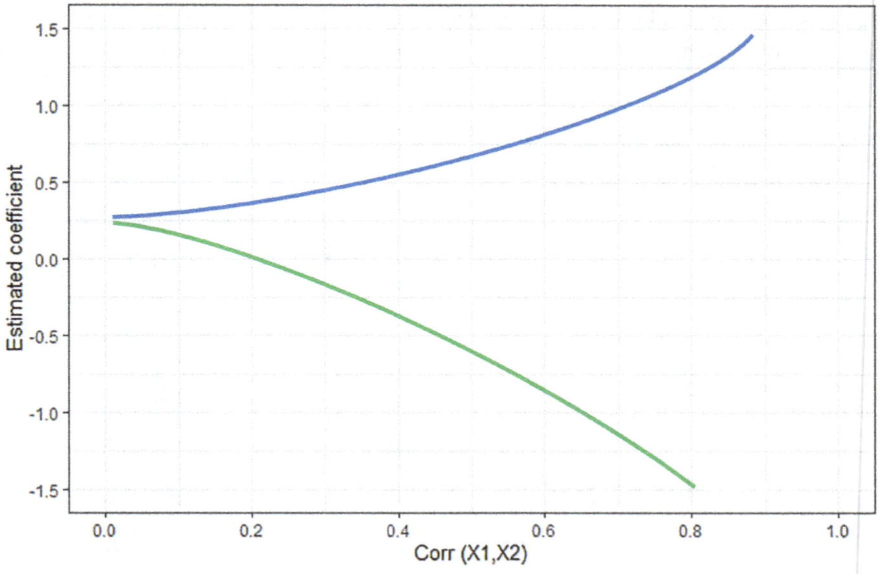

Fig. 3.3 The reversal paradox: parameter estimates of two highly correlated predictors will often tend to inflate in opposite directions when mutually included in a regression model

This issue is commonly known as the *reversal paradox*, occurring when the parameter estimates of two correlated covariates inflate in opposite directions. Of note, high correlation does not necessarily imply that results will be affected by collinearity, but rather increases the risk that collinearity might be present. In some situations, coefficients could present extreme levels of inflation, as observed, for example, by Chiu et al. [6]. There are other settings, however, where applying multiple regression on correlated data could provided reliable results that are then confirmed by more robust approaches [3]. This is often the case when the association between each correlated exposure and the outcome is either null or relatively weak.

To quantify the severity of multicollinearity in a regression analysis, one should calculate the *variance inflation factor* (VIF). VIFs are calculated for each predictor in a regression model and provide a measure of how much the variance of that estimated regression coefficient is increased because of collinearity. Higher VIFs indicate that those coefficients are likely affected by the high correlations between the corresponding predictor and other covariates in the model. In practical situations, VIFs values as low as 4 or 5 should already set the alarm off. Table 3.3 shows VIFs in our illustrative example, confirming that the results for correlated exposures are heavily affected by multicollinearity.

Collinearity is not the only potential problem that can arise when applying multiple regression in the context of environmental mixtures. In particular, even in the presence of low levels of correlations, the inclusion of several covariates in the same regression model might increase the risk of *model overfitting*. This threat gets increasingly more important as additional assumptions of non-linearity and non-additivity are also relaxed. The concept of overfitting and alternative approaches that can be considered in complex settings will be the the focus of Chap. 5. The next

Table 3.3 Variance inflation factors (VIFs) of regression coefficients from multiple regression (Table 3.2) in the NHANES data

	VIF
X_1	1.236
X_2	1.318
X_3	49.480
X_4	58.242
X_5	11.256
X_6	2.271
X_7	2.723
X_8	3.893
X_9	2.553
X_{10}	2.811
X_{11}	3.694
X_{12}	6.086
X_{13}	6.557
X_{14}	3.152
Z_1	1.140
Z_2	4.784
Z_3	1.135

section will instead describe the statistical framework of penalized regression, which directly addresses the problem of collinearity and is, as such, of particular importance for the assessment of mixture-health associations.

3.3 Penalized Regression

Penalization is a powerful statistical tool to address some of the challenges that arise when building regression models with many variables. Penalized regression models can be described as extensions of standard regression models where a *penalty* factor is incorporated in the loss function. The appeal of penalized regression in the context of assessing mixture-health associations is due to the fact that this penalization procedure targets the *variance* of the model and it tends to decrease the influence of collinearity in the presence of high levels of correlations between covariates. The price we pay for this decrease in model variability is the introduction of some *bias* to the parameter estimates. Specifically, the penalization will shrink coefficients toward zero, the reason why these approaches are also referred to as *shrinkage* methods.

3.3.1 *Bias-Variance Trade-Off*

The word *bias* will mostly trigger negative reactions to the trained environmental epidemiologist [9, 14, 16]. To fully appreciate the advantages of penalized regression, it is therefore useful to provide some additional details on what bias means in this context and how this penalization is implemented.

The goal of a linear regression model is to predict n observations of the response variable, Y, with a linear combination of p predictor variables, X, and a normally distributed error term with variance σ^2:

$$Y = \beta_0 + \sum_{i=1}^{p} \beta_i \cdot X_i + \beta \cdot C\epsilon, \tag{3.3}$$

with $\epsilon \sim N(0, \sigma^2)$.

A rule to estimate the parameters β from the sample is required, and a standard choice to do so is by using *ordinary least square* (OLS), which produce estimates $\hat{\beta}$ by minimizing the sum of squares of residuals. Specifically, OLS minimizes the following *loss function*:

$$L_{OLS}(\hat{\beta}) = \sum_{i=1}^{n} (y_i - x_i'\hat{\beta})^2 = \|y - X\hat{\beta}\|^2 \tag{3.4}$$

Using matrix notation, the OLS estimate of the parameters can be expressed as

$$\hat{\beta}_{OLS} = (X'X)^{-1}(X'Y) \tag{3.5}$$

To evaluate the performance of an estimator, there are two critical characteristics to be considered: its *bias* and its *variance*. The bias of an estimator measures the *accuracy* of the estimates:

$$Bias(\hat{\beta}_{OLS}) = E(\hat{\beta}_{OLS}) - \beta \tag{3.6}$$

The variance, on the other hand, measures the *uncertainty* of the estimates:

$$Var(\hat{\beta}_{OLS}) = \sigma^2(X'X)^{-1} \tag{3.7}$$

An intuitive example to illustrate the ideas of bias and variance of an estimator is to think of it as an Olympic archer (Fig. 3.4). The best athlete is the archer (estimator) with low bias and low variance (middle panel), who consistently hits the target with high levels of precision. An archer (estimator) with low bias but high variance has less precision, but, on average, hits around the center (right panel). Nevertheless, each individual shot (the estimate in a specific population) will likely be off. On the opposite side of the spectrum (left panel), we have the archer (estimator) with high bias and low variance, who is extremely precise in consistently shooting at the wrong target. The main property of the OLS estimator is that it is asymptotically *unbiased*. Using the archery example, OLS always ends up in either

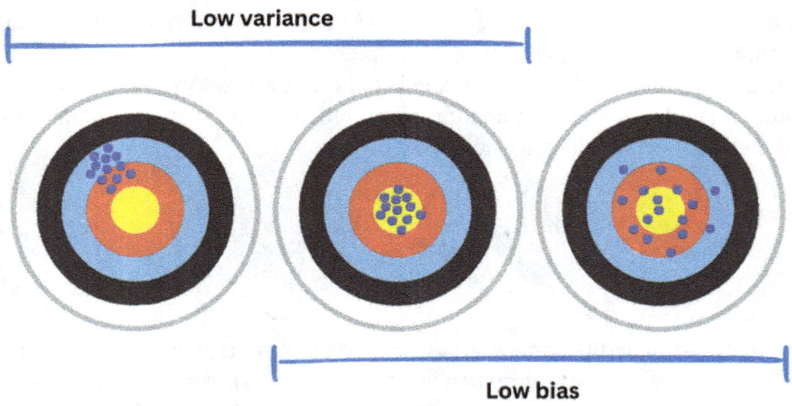

Fig. 3.4 The OLS estimator is asymptotically unbiased. As such it behaves like an Olympic archer who, on average, hits the bull's eye (middle or right panels). At higher levels of model complexity, however, the estimator's variance will increase, and the performance of OLS will more likely resemble those of the archer on the right

the center or right situation. The likelihood to which OLS will move to settings of high variance is related to the level of model complexity. One of these situations, in particular, is the one where the model is affected by collinearity.

When high variance is of potential threat, a better way to assess the performance of the model is to take into account both bias and variance. Specifically, we use the mean squared error (MSE), defined as the sum of variance and squared bias:

$$MSE = \frac{1}{n}\sum_{i=1}^{n}(Y_i - \hat{Y}_i)^2 = Var(\hat{\beta}) + Bias^2(\hat{\beta}) \tag{3.8}$$

The general idea of *bias-variance trade-off* is to introduce some bias in order to minimize the MSE, thus improving the performance of the estimator in those situations where high variance will affect OLS performances. This trade-off is achieved by augmenting the loss function in Eq. 3.4 through the introduction of a penalty. The next subsections will describe the three more common choices for a penalty function and the corresponding regression models, Ridge, LASSO, and Elastic Net regression, with the latter being a generalized version of the previous two.

3.3.2 Ridge

Ridge regression augments the OLS loss function by penalizing the size of the parameter estimates, shrinking them toward zero:

$$L_{ridge}(\hat{\beta}) = \sum_{i=1}^{n}(y_i - x_i'\hat{\beta})^2 + \lambda\sum_{j=1}^{m}\hat{\beta}_j^2 = \|y - X\hat{\beta}\|^2 + \lambda\|\hat{\beta}\|^2 \tag{3.9}$$

The new parameter λ represents the penalty factor and indicates the level of shrinkage that has to be operated. As $\lambda \to 0$, $\hat{\beta}_{ridge} \to \hat{\beta}_{OLS}$, while as $\lambda \to \infty$, $\hat{\beta}_{ridge} \to 0$. In words, setting λ to 0 will reduce Ridge to the standard OLS. Higher levels of λ, on the other hand, will provide stronger penalization. The unique feature of Ridge regression, as compared to other penalization techniques, is that this shrinking of the coefficients will only reach 0 asymptotically. In practice, this implies that all covariates will always be retained in the model for any level of λ. Figure 3.5 shows the trajectory of estimated coefficients in the NHANES illustrative data at increasing levels of the Ridge penalty factor. The numbers displayed on top of the figure indicate the number of coefficients retained in the model, which will always correspond to the original number of predictors in the case of Ridge.

The key question in penalized regression is how much one is willing to trade, or, more technically, how to identify the optimal level of λ. Out of several approaches,

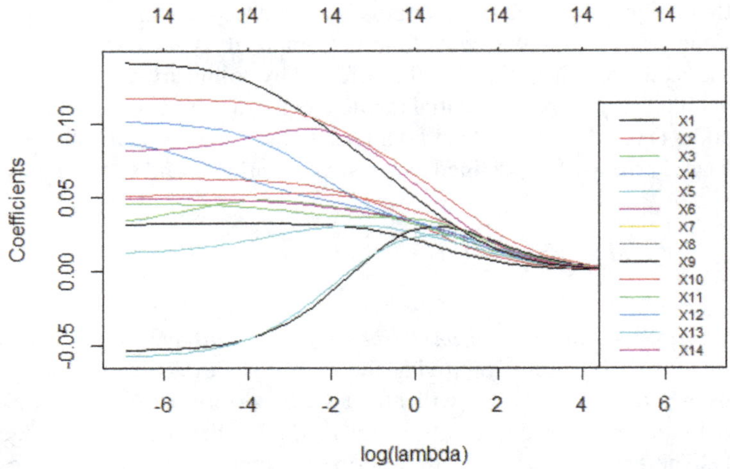

Fig. 3.5 Trajectory of regression coefficients for Ridge regression in the NHANES dataset

a robust procedure based on cross-validation is recommended in most settings as it also addresses the problem of overfitting.[3] The reader can refer to the software material available on the accompanying Github page (https://github.com/andreabellavia/statsmixtures) for details on how to implement this cross-validation procedure in R (packages `glmnet` and `coxnet`). An accurate description of this λ selection procedure in an applied setting can be found in Lenters et al. [12], which provides a thorough application of penalized regression for environmental mixtures.

Figure 3.6 presents the MSE as a function of λ when fitting Ridge regression on the NHANES illustrative data. The vertical dashed lines correspond to the λ that minimize MSE and the cross-validated λ. Results from the model using the optimal λ as inferred from cross-validation are presented in Table 3.4. This table provides some comforting results as we do not see any negative coefficients anymore, effectively proving that the model choice has likely addressed collinearity issues. At the same time, the shrinking of the coefficients does not provide substantial information in terms of who the bad actors within the mixture could be. For example, members of the highly correlated group $X_3 - X_5$ are roughly given the same estimate. For this reason, when studying environmental mixtures, alternative penalties might be preferred to the Ridge one. In particular, the choice generally falls on the LASSO or the Elastic Net penalties, which also provide a form of *variable selection*.

[3] Additional details on cross-validation and its relationship to overfitting are provided in Sect. 5.4.1.

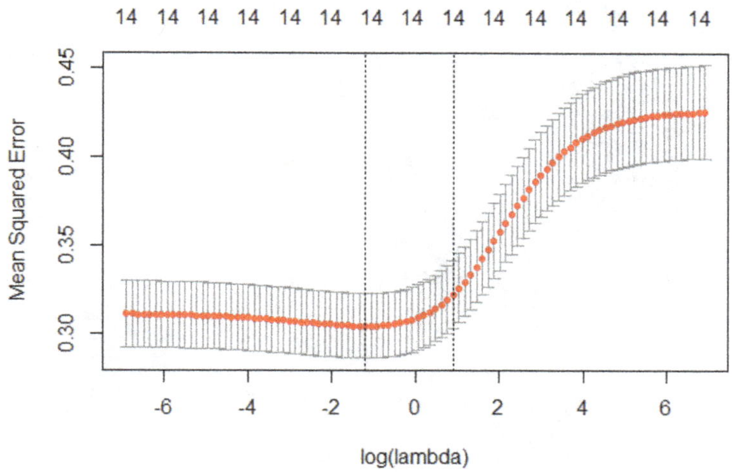

Fig. 3.6 Mean squared error as a function of Ridge penalty factor in the NHANES dataset

Table 3.4 Ridge regression: parameter estimates in the NHANES dataset

	Estimate
X_1	0.013
X_2	0.021
X_3	0.024
X_4	0.025
X_5	0.020
X_6	0.026
X_7	0.029
X_8	0.031
X_9	0.030
X_{10}	0.026
X_{11}	0.024
X_{12}	0.038
X_{13}	0.032
X_{14}	0.047

3.3.3 LASSO

The Least Absolute Shrinkage and Selection Operator (LASSO), rather than penalizing by the sum of squared residuals as in Eq. 3.9, penalizes the loss function of OLS by the sum of their absolute values:

$$L_{lasso}(\hat{\beta}) = \sum_{i=1}^{n}(y_i - x_i'\hat{\beta})^2 + \lambda \sum_{j=1}^{m} |\hat{\beta}_j| \tag{3.10}$$

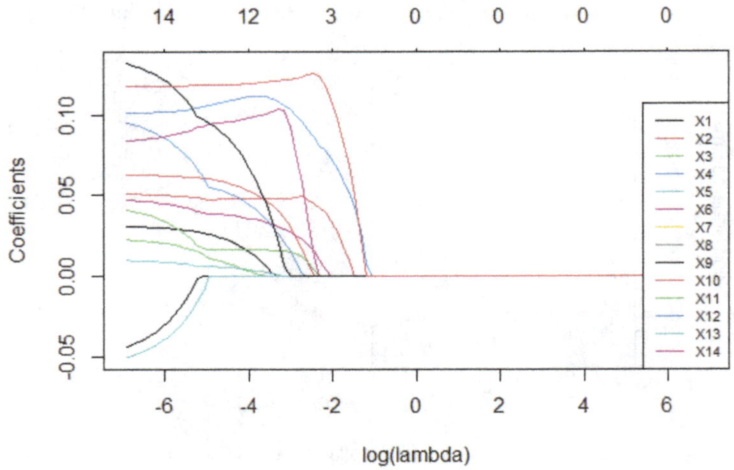

Fig. 3.7 Trajectory of regression coefficients for LASSO regression in the NHANES dataset

As a results, while the Ridge shrinking was only pushing coefficients to 0 asymptotically, the LASSO procedure will result in several coefficients being exactly zeroed at high levels of λ. Figure 3.7 shows the trajectory of regression coefficients when applying LASSO to the NHANES illustrative data. As indicated by the numbers displayed on top of the figure, the model selects a smaller number of covariates at higher shrinkage levels.

The selection of the optimal value for λ is conducted using the same cross-validation approach as for Ridge and is presented, for this illustrative example, in Fig. 3.8. Results from LASSO regression using the selected λ are instead presented in Table 3.5. Only four covariates are retained in this final model: X_4, X_6, X_8, X_{14}. This is certainly a significant improvement as we are capturing three of the main real predictors. At the same time, this comes at the expense of several additional risk factors (e.g., X_{12}) that are left out. This is not unexpected. LASSO's results, in general, tend to be very sensitive to weak associations, dropping coefficients that are not actually 0, and it usually performs better when there is a small number of significant parameters with all others close to zero (i.e., when only a few predictors actually influence the outcome).

3.3.4 Elastic Net

Elastic Net has been designed as a compromise between LASSO and Ridge, attempting to overcome their limitations and performing variable selection in a less rigid way than LASSO. Elastic Net combines the penalties of Ridge regression and LASSO, aiming at minimizing the following loss function:

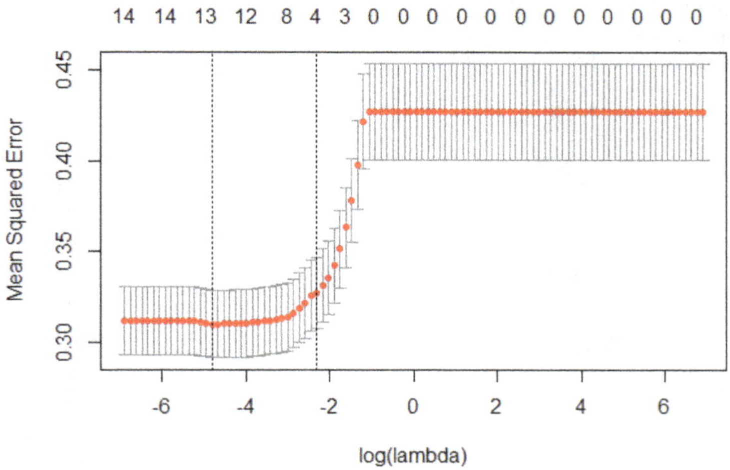

Fig. 3.8 Mean squared error as a function of LASSO penalty factor in the NHANES dataset

Table 3.5 LASSO regression: parameter estimates in the NHANES dataset

	Estimate
X_1	/
X_2	/
X_3	/
X_4	0.080
X_5	/
X_6	0.009
X_7	/
X_8	0.041
X_9	/
X_{10}	/
X_{11}	/
X_{12}	/
X_{13}	/
X_{14}	0.122

$$L_{enet}(\hat{\beta}) = \frac{\sum_{i=1}^{n}(y_i - x_i'\hat{\beta})^2}{2n} + \lambda\left(\frac{1-\alpha}{2}\sum_{j=1}^{m}\hat{\beta}_j^2 + \alpha\sum_{j=1}^{m}|\hat{\beta}_j|\right) \tag{3.11}$$

where α is the mixing parameter between Ridge ($\alpha = 0$) and LASSO ($\alpha = 1$). How this loss function is derived, given the Ridge and LASSO ones, is described in Zou et al. [25]. Procedures to simultaneously tune both α and λ to retrieve the optimal combinations are available and integrated in the R package `caret`. Table 3.6 includes results from fitting Elastic Net regression in the NHANES dataset.

Table 3.6 Elastic Net regression: parameter estimates in the NHANES dataset

	Estimate
X_1	/
X_2	/
X_3	0.021
X_4	0.049
X_5	0.010
X_6	0.017
X_7	/
X_8	0.045
X_9	0.004
X_{10}	/
X_{11}	/
X_{12}	/
X_{13}	/
X_{14}	0.116

As expected, less covariates are dropped to 0. The relaxed penalty, however, reintroduces some noise for those covariates that are not truly associated with the outcome but present high levels of correlations with real predictors (e.g., X_3 and X_5).[4] This is an expected result due to specific properties of Elastic Net vs LASSO: specifically, within a group of highly correlated covariates, LASSO tends to only select one variable, while Elastic Net is more likely to retrieve most of the cluster members.

3.3.5 *Practical Notes and Relevant Extensions*

Confounding Control in Penalized Regression
Penalized regression techniques allow controlling for potential confounders, which can be done by specifying them as additional covariates in the model as in a regular GLM. When applying penalized regression to environmental mixtures, however, we generally do not want confounders to be included in the selection process. All R packages allow informing the cross-validation procedure that the shrinkage should only happen for mixture components, while coefficients for confounders should remain untouched.

Replicate Results with GLM
When LASSO or Elastic Net are used to describe associations in population-based studies, it is common practice to also present a final linear regression model that

[4] Note that these results are subject to the specific choice and tuning procedure operated for λ and α.

only includes those predictors that were selected from the penalized approach [12]. This two-step approach will ensure a robust selection of relevant predictors, via penalized regression, and a better interpretation of the coefficients via GLM to provide unbiased estimates. When this approach is chosen, however, caution must be taken on the interpretation of p-values and standard errors from the final GLM model, which are calculated without taking into account that variable selection has been operated in a previous step.

Adaptive Grouped LASSO
There are several settings where mixture components can be classified to some specific subgroups, whether pre-defined or identified from unsupervised approaches such as PCA. This grouping information can be used to improve the shrinkage and selection procedure operated by LASSO with the use of the grouped LASSO extensions [5, 21]. A specific extension of this approach, namely, adaptive grouped LASSO, is preferred in most cases to avoid issues of selection inconsistency commonly observed with grouped LASSO [20, 24].

3.4 Penalized Regression: Concluding Remarks

Penalized regression approaches, and in particular LASSO and Elastic Net, represent a robust framework for the assessment of exposure-health associations, as documented by the several applications presented in the literature (see, e.g., [2, 11, 12, 19, 22]). Several review papers have confirmed the robustness of this tool as compared to both alternative regression-based approaches and modern methods [1, 10]. In this context, it is important to understand the specific advantages and limitations of regression-based approaches to better appreciate the need of additional techniques and to identify those settings where alternative methodologies should be considered.

The main advantage of penalized regression is the ability to conduct variable selection by taking into account the potentially complex levels of correlation between the different predictors. This can provide robust conclusions about the identification of the *bad actors* within the environmental mixture. As discussed in Sect. 1.3, however, this is only one of the several research questions that researchers might be interested in when assessing the health effects of environmental mixtures.

Assessing the Cumulative Mixture Effect
LASSO and Elastic Net address the issues of collinearity and high-dimensionality by operating a shrinkage procedure that result in some sort of variable selection. While this allows retrieving information on individual effects for a selected component, it also prevents addressing questions on what the *cumulative (overall) effect* of the mixture is. This is a research question with relevant public health implications. Methods discussed in the next chapter address the complexity of the mixture through indexing rather than variable selection, thus improving the estimation of this cumulative effect measure.

Complex Settings
When the mixture of interest is composed of several environmental factors, it is likely that complex mechanisms will be involved in generating the mixture-health effects. For example, as the number of potential predictors increases, so does the chance that non-linear and non-additive effects will be present. With several covariates at play, however, incorporating non-linear and non-additive effects in GLM and penalized regression is not straightforward. Chapter 5 will discuss these limitations in details and introduce alternative modeling techniques that can take into account such data complexities.

References

1. Lydiane Agier, Lützen Portengen, Marc Chadeau-Hyam, Xavier Basagaña, Lise Giorgis-Allemand, Valérie Siroux, Oliver Robinson, Jelle Vlaanderen, Juan R González, Mark J Nieuwenhuijsen, et al. A systematic comparison of linear regression–based statistical methods to assess exposome-health associations. *Environmental health perspectives*, 124(12):1848–1856, 2016.
2. Max T Aung, Youfei Yu, Kelly K Ferguson, David E Cantonwine, Lixia Zeng, Thomas F McElrath, Subramaniam Pennathur, Bhramar Mukherjee, and John D Meeker. Cross-sectional estimation of endogenous biomarker associations with prenatal phenols, phthalates, metals, and polycyclic aromatic hydrocarbons in single-pollutant and mixtures analysis approaches. *Environmental health perspectives*, 129(3):037007, 2021.
3. Andrea Bellavia, Yu-Han Chiu, Florence M Brown, Lidia Mínguez-Alarcón, Jennifer B Ford, Myra Keller, John Petrozza, Paige L Williams, Xiaoyun Ye, Antonia M Calafat, et al. Urinary concentrations of parabens mixture and pregnancy glucose levels among women from a fertility clinic. *Environmental research*, 168:389–396, 2019.
4. Cécile Billionnet, Duane Sherrill, Isabella Annesi-Maesano, et al. Estimating the health effects of exposure to multi-pollutant mixture. *Annals of epidemiology*, 22(2):126–141, 2012.
5. Jonathan Boss, Alexander Rix, Yin-Hsiu Chen, Naveen N Narisetty, Zhenke Wu, Kelly K Ferguson, Thomas F McElrath, John D Meeker, and Bhramar Mukherjee. A hierarchical integrative group least absolute shrinkage and selection operator for analyzing environmental mixtures. *Environmetrics*, 32(8):e2698, 2021.
6. Yu-Han Chiu, Andrea Bellavia, Tamarra James-Todd, Katharine F Correia, Linda Valeri, Carmen Messerlian, Jennifer B Ford, Lidia Mínguez-Alarcón, Antonia M Calafat, Russ Hauser, et al. Evaluating effects of prenatal exposure to phthalate mixtures on birth weight: A comparison of three statistical approaches. *Environment international*, 113:231–239, 2018.
7. Jean C Digitale, Jeffrey N Martin, and Medellena Maria Glymour. Tutorial on directed acyclic graphs. *Journal of Clinical Epidemiology*, 142:264–267, 2022.
8. Francesca Dominici, Roger D Peng, Christopher D Barr, and Michelle L Bell. Protecting human health from air pollution: shifting from a single-pollutant to a multipollutant approach. *Epidemiology*, 21(2):187–194, 2010.
9. Stephanie M Eick, Dana E Goin, Nicholas Chartres, Juleen Lam, and Tracey J Woodruff. Assessing risk of bias in human environmental epidemiology studies using three tools: different conclusions from different tools. *Systematic reviews*, 9:1–13, 2020.
10. Elizabeth A Gibson, Yanelli Nunez, Ahlam Abuawad, Ami R Zota, Stefano Renzetti, Katrina L Devick, Chris Gennings, Jeff Goldsmith, Brent A Coull, and Marianthi-Anna Kioumourtzoglou. An overview of methods to address distinct research questions on environmental mixtures: an application to persistent organic pollutants and leukocyte telomere length. *Environmental Health*, 18:1–16, 2019.

11. Jie Hu, George D Papandonatos, Tongzhang Zheng, Joseph M Braun, Bin Zhang, Wenyu Liu, Chuansha Wu, Aifen Zhou, Simin Liu, Stephen L Buka, et al. Prenatal metal mixture exposure and birth weight: A two-stage analysis in two prospective cohort studies. *Eco-Environment & Health*, 1(3):165–171, 2022.
12. Virissa Lenters, Lützen Portengen, Anna Rignell-Hydbom, Bo AG Jönsson, Christian H Lindh, Aldert H Piersma, Gunnar Toft, Jens Peter Bonde, Dick Heederik, Lars Rylander, et al. Prenatal phthalate, perfluoroalkyl acid, and organochlorine exposures and term birth weight in three birth cohorts: multi-pollutant models based on elastic net regression. *Environmental health perspectives*, 124(3):365–372, 2016.
13. Chirag J Patel, Jayanta Bhattacharya, and Atul J Butte. An environment-wide association study (ewas) on type 2 diabetes mellitus. *PloS one*, 5(5):e10746, 2010.
14. Juha Pekkanen and Neil Pearce. Environmental epidemiology: challenges and opportunities. *Environmental health perspectives*, 109(1):1–5, 2001.
15. Roger D Peng and Francesca Dominici. Statistical methods for environmental epidemiology with R. *R: a case study in air pollution and health*, 2008.
16. Kenneth J Rothman. Methodologic frontiers in environmental epidemiology. *Environmental health perspectives*, 101(suppl 4):19–21, 1993.
17. Kyla W Taylor, Bonnie R Joubert, Joe M Braun, Caroline Dilworth, Chris Gennings, Russ Hauser, Jerry J Heindel, Cynthia V Rider, Thomas F Webster, and Danielle J Carlin. Statistical approaches for assessing health effects of environmental chemical mixtures in epidemiology: lessons from an innovative workshop. *Environmental health perspectives*, 124(12):A227–A229, 2016.
18. Duncan C Thomas. *Statistical methods in environmental epidemiology*. OUP Oxford, 2009.
19. Annette Vriens, Tim S Nawrot, Willy Baeyens, Elly Den Hond, Liesbeth Bruckers, Adrian Covaci, Kim Croes, Sam De Craemer, Eva Govarts, Nathalie Lambrechts, et al. Neonatal exposure to environmental pollutants and placental mitochondrial dna content: a multi-pollutant approach. *Environment international*, 106:60–68, 2017.
20. Hansheng Wang and Chenlei Leng. A note on adaptive group lasso. *Computational statistics & data analysis*, 52(12):5277–5286, 2008.
21. Ming Yuan and Yi Lin. Model selection and estimation in regression with grouped variables. *Journal of the Royal Statistical Society Series B: Statistical Methodology*, 68(1):49–67, 2006.
22. Hao Zhao, Jun Tang, Qinheng Zhu, Hongsen He, Shuai Li, Lanfei Jin, Xue Zhang, Longtao Zhu, Jing Guo, Dan Zhang, et al. Associations of prenatal heavy metals exposure with placental characteristics and birth weight in hangzhou birth cohort: Multi-pollutant models based on elastic net regression. *Science of The Total Environment*, 742:140613, 2020.
23. Yi Zheng, Zhaoyi Chen, Thomas Pearson, Jinying Zhao, Hui Hu, and Mattia Prosperi. Design and methodology challenges of environment-wide association studies: A systematic review. *Environmental research*, 183:109275, 2020.
24. Yinnan Zheng, Cuilin Zhang, Marc G Weisskopf, Paige L Williams, Birgit Claus Henn, Patrick J Parsons, Christopher D Palmer, Germaine M Buck Louis, and Tamarra James-Todd. Evaluating associations between early pregnancy trace elements mixture and 2nd trimester gestational glucose levels: A comparison of three statistical approaches. *International journal of hygiene and environmental health*, 224:113446, 2020.
25. Hui Zou and Trevor Hastie. Regularization and variable selection via the elastic net. *Journal of the royal statistical society: series B (statistical methodology)*, 67(2):301–320, 2005.

Chapter 4
Mixture Indexing Approaches

4.1 Introduction to Indexing

The previous chapter introduced the use of regression modeling to assess the association between an environmental mixture and a health outcome. Exploiting the use of established and familiar frameworks such as generalized linear modeling and penalized regression was the natural starting point when the field of environmental epidemiology began the transition from a single-pollutant to a multi-pollutant approach. As discussed in Chap. 3, extensions of classical regressions can account for several of the complexities of environmental mixtures and should be considered, at least as a first analytical step, in applied research. At the same time, some of the unique challenges associated with assessing the health effects of environmental mixtures have motivated researchers to develop ad hoc statistical methodologies that can address the specific complexities of the field. A statistical tool that has been widely employed to this extent is the concept of *indexing*. The first subsection of this chapter will describe the general idea of indexing and introduce intuitive approaches for unsupervised indexing in environmental epidemiology. The second part of the chapter will instead discuss supervised indexing approaches with specific focus on Weighted Quantile Sum (WQS) regression and its extensions.

In statistics, indexing refers to the use of a series of values to create a single summary number. Applications of indexing are ubiquitous in clinical and epidemiological research. In clinical research, for example, *risk scores* are developed to summarize the individual risk of a given health outcome based on several covariates [49]. The same concept is also applied in genomics where *polygenic risk scores* are used to summarize with a single number the individual risk of a given medical condition based on a full genome-wide assessment [31]. In epidemiology, an example of an indexing technique is the *propensity score*, which is used to summarize individual profiles of several potential confounders for a more robust assessment of causal effects [1]. Indexing approaches also sit at the core of the development of *latent factors*, especially common in psychology, where a set of

A. Bellavia, *Statistical Methods for Environmental Mixtures*, Society, Environment and Statistics, https://doi.org/10.1007/978-3-031-78987-8_4

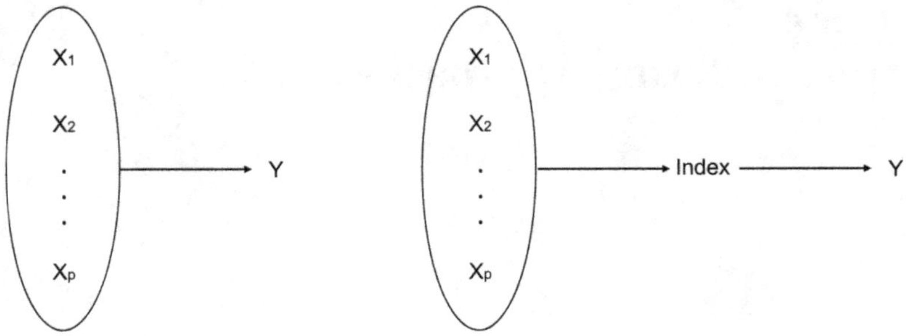

Fig. 4.1 General idea of mixture indexing: rather than directly assessing the effects of each predictor (left), the mixture is summarized into a single score that is then evaluated as a predictor of health (right)

observed variables are used to estimate the value of a single unobserved (latent) variable [3].

In the context of environmental mixtures, the idea of indexing can be used to summarize individual levels of exposure to the mixture of interest into a single summary score. This index can then be used in a regression model replacing the several original exposures with the summary index, as illustratively displayed in Fig. 4.1.

Including a summary index in a regression model provides considerable modeling advantages. Using the NHANES illustrative data example, we discussed how including all 14 covariates in a single regression model as in Eq. 4.1 would introduce severe issues due to collinearity and overfitting:

$$Y_i = \beta_0 + \beta_1 \cdot X_{1i} + \beta_2 \cdot X_{2i} + \cdots + \beta_{14} \cdot X_{14i} + \epsilon_i \tag{4.1}$$

A mixture indexing approach would allow identifying an individual value $index_i$ that can comprehensively summarize the exposure profile of individual i to the 14 mixture components. We could then replace model 4.1 with model 4.2, which only contains one covariate and is not anymore subject to the discussed limitations:

$$Y_i = \alpha_0 + \alpha_1 \cdot index_i + \epsilon_i \tag{4.2}$$

Model 4.2 does not directly incorporate the specific mixture components, thus precluding the estimation of exposure-specific effects. However, the new parameter α_1 has the key interpretation of a *cumulative mixture effect*. This is a single parameter that can be used to summarize the overall effect of exposure to the mixture of interest, with considerable advantages in terms of translating results into potential public health recommendations.

The key for model 4.2 to be of practical utility is whether the index really represents a reliable and robust summary of individual exposures. There are several ways a mixture index can be calculated, which we can broadly categorize into unsupervised and supervised approaches.

4.2 Unsupervised Summary Scores

Unsupervised summary scores attempt to describe individual profiles of exposure without accounting for any specific exposure-outcome relationship. In practice, analyses under this approach are conducted in two stages: first, a summary index is calculated; next, the index is included in a statistical model such as 4.2 to assess the association between the index (the cumulative mixture exposure) and the outcome. There are some common examples of unsupervised scores widely used in environmental epidemiology.

Weighted Aggregation of Specific Chemical Subgroups (Molar Sum)
Aggregation techniques are often selected for a specific subgroup of environmental chemicals with similar biology and possibly extreme levels of correlation. This is the standard approach, for example, to investigate DEHP metabolites [8]. Specimen samples used to assess phthalates metabolites will often provide individual concentrations of at least four common DEHP metabolites, which are usually complicated to disentangle in statistical analysis due to their extreme levels of correlations (e.g., >0.9) [26]. A solution is to aggregate these metabolites using their *molar sum*, commonly referred to as $\sum$ DEHP. To fairly incorporate the potential differences in molecular mass between metabolites, the sum is calculated by weighting each metabolite for their molecular weights [21]. In applied settings, this aggregation is often conducted as a preliminary step before any statistical analysis, directly assessing $\sum$ DEHP as a covariate of interest or as a specific component of a wider phthalate mixture (see, e.g., [22]). The implicit consequence of this approach is that results will not be able to capture the specific contribution of each DEHP metabolite in determining a given exposure-outcome association. Despite being used less frequently than the $\sum$ DEHP, additional molar sums have been used to describe other subgroups of metabolites (see, e.g.,[44, 53]).

Principal Components and Latent Variables
As discussed in Sec. 2.4, results from PCA are sometimes integrated in a regression model to summarize specific subgroups of exposures (see, e.g., [35, 48]). The appeal of this approach is that principal components are uncorrelated by design, thus implicitly addressing any problem of collinearity. A severe limitation of this approach, however, is that such a regression model will only account for the proportion of the mixture variability explained by the included components.[1] Moreover, a meaningful biological/chemical interpretation of the extracted components is critical for the results of the regression model to be interpretable. Application of regression modeling with principal components can be found, among others, in Lee et al. [28] and Sanchez et al. [45].

---

[1] As discussed in Sec. 2.4, from a starting set of p covariates, it would take p components to summarize all the variability. We generally select components that explain about 70–80 %.

4.3 Weighted Quantile Sum (WQS) Regression

Weighted Quantile Sum (WQS) regression was first introduced in 2015 [5, 12] and has since become one of the most popular and widely used approaches for the assessment of mixture-health associations in environmental epidemiology. Specifically, WQS regression is a statistical approach where exposure aggregation via indexing is conducted in a supervised fashion within the assessment of the mixture-outcome association. In practice, the two steps previously described of i) creating a summary index and ii) including the index in a regression model are now conducted within the same statistical estimation procedure. Because of this supervised nature, within the same dataset and the same set of environmental exposures, WQS regression would derive different indexes when assessing the association between the original mixture and different health outcomes. Unsupervised approaches, on the other hand, would use the same summary index for any outcome.

WQS owes its name to three important properties involved in the definition of the summary index:

- Weighted. First, the index is constructed by *weighting* each mixture component. The previously described molar sums weigh each exposure by their molecular weight. WQS, instead, weights each exposure by how much it contributes to the overall mixture-outcome association.
- Quantile. Second, the index is not directly built on the mixture components but rather on their transformations into categorical exposures based on some *quantiles* of their distributions. Often, this categorization is based on quartiles (four levels) or deciles (ten levels) of the exposure distributions.
- Sum. Third, the index is built as a weighted *linear sum* of the exposures. For each subject, the value of the index will be determined by summing up the individual levels of exposure to the mixture component, each weighted by the estimated weights.

A WQS regression model takes the following form:

$$f(y) = \beta_0 + \beta_1\left(\sum_{i=1}^{p} w_i q_i\right) + \beta \cdot C \tag{4.3}$$

where $f(y)$ is a transformation of the outcome of interest[2] and C is a vector of potential confounders. The linear sum $\sum_{i=1}^{p} w_i q_i$ is the index (the weighted quantile sum), with q_i representing the p categorical transformations of the original exposures X_i, each weighted by w_i. These weights are unknown and are treated as parameters to be estimated by the model. The basic formulation of WQS regression is an extension of GLM, and the β parameters will therefore hold the

[2] Possible modeling includes linear, logistic, multinomial, Poisson, and negative binomial regression.

classical GLM interpretations. Specifically, $\hat{\beta}_1$ can be interpreted as the overall (or cumulative) effect of the mixture. The specific interpretation of this coefficient is not straightforward. As described, exposures are categorized into quantiles of their distributions and aggregated as a weighted sum. Therefore, $\hat{\beta}_1$ represents the expected change in $f(y)$ (e.g., the average of Y for a continuous outcome, the log(OR) for a binary outcome) when all exposures jointly change from one quantile to the next.[3]

4.3.1 Estimation

Parameter estimation is commonly conducted by splitting the dataset into a training and a validation set: the first set is used for the weight estimation, while the second one is used to test for the significance of the final WQS index. A common approach is to use a 40/60 ratio, but alternative splits can be explored. The weights are estimated using bootstrap[4] and subject to two constraints: to be bounded between 0 and 1 ($0 \leq w_i \leq 1$) and to sum up to 1 ($\sum_{i=1}^{c} w_i = 1$). These constraints allow interpreting the weights as estimating the relative importance of each exposure in the observed cumulative effect.

For each bootstrap sample (at least 100 bootstrap sample replications are recommended), weights are estimated through an optimization algorithm [18] as described in Czarnota et al. [12]. When averaging the estimates across bootstrap samples, another important assumption is introduced. Specifically, WQS makes an assumption of *unidirectionality*. The user has to define a priori whether to estimate a positive or a negative effect. Such effect will then be calculated only including component-specific contributions in the pre-specified direction. For example, the effect of the mixture in the positive direction will be estimated as a (weighted) cumulative effect of the positive effects of each mixture component. Vice versa, the negative effect will be estimated as a (weighted) cumulative effect of the negative effects of each mixture component. This assumption is implemented by only averaging results over bootstrap samples with either positive or negative estimates.

Specifically, the final estimate of the WQS will be calculated as weighted sum of the p components as

---

[3] This basic formulation also makes a linearity assumption for the index where the effect is assumed to be the same for each quantile change. For example, if four categories were used based on distribution quartiles, β_1 would represent the effect when all exposures change from the first to the second quartile, from the second to the third, or from the third to the fourth.

[4] Bootstrap is a procedure for estimating the distribution of an estimator of interest via sampling with replacement of the same dataset. For a gentle introduction to bootstrap, see, for example, Rousselet et al. [43].

$$WQS = \sum_{i=1}^{c} \bar{w}_i q_i \tag{4.4}$$

where $\overline{w}_i = \frac{1}{n_B}\sum_{h=1}^{n_B} w_{ih}$, with n_B being the number of bootstrap samples where the estimate of β_1 was either positive or negative. This final estimate of the WQS is used to fit model 4.3 in the validation set to obtain the estimates of the remaining β parameters.

4.3.2 Results Interpretations and Practical Considerations

Software Implementation
WQS is fully implemented in the R package gWQS (standing for *generalized* WQS). R codes to replicate results presented in this section, together with links to the extensive online material describing the package, are provided in the accompanying web page (https://github.com/andreabellavia/statsmixtures).

User-Defined Options
When fitting a WQS regression model, the following options have to be selected by the user:

- Training/validation ratio
- Number of bootstrap samples
- Number of quantiles for the exposure categorization

In practical applications it is recommended to check whether results are robust to different tuning of all these options. Additionally and most importantly, the user has to select whether a positive or negative model should be estimated. It is always recommended to assess the model in both directions as this could provide insights of the specific contribution of each mixture component as they affect the outcome (see, e.g., the WQS results presentation in Deyssenroth et al. [14]).

Results Interpretation
Figure 4.2 presents the estimates of the weights after fitting a WQS regression model with positive directionality assumption in the NHANES illustrative data, using quartiles for exposure categorization and 100 bootstrap samples with a 40/60 training-validation split. The estimate of β_1 is 0.27 (95% CI: 0.23–0.32), indicating the presence of a positive effect of the mixture on the outcome Y. The figure displays the ranking of exposures as they contribute to this overall effect. All relevant predictors are given substantial weight, and the model is also correctly identifying the top predictors in X_6, X_1, and X_{12}, which are all given weights over 10%. Of note, these results are correctly capturing X_4 as the most important component within the group of correlated exposures $X_3 - X_5$, and X_{12} as the important contributor between the other correlated cluster $X_{12} - X_{13}$.

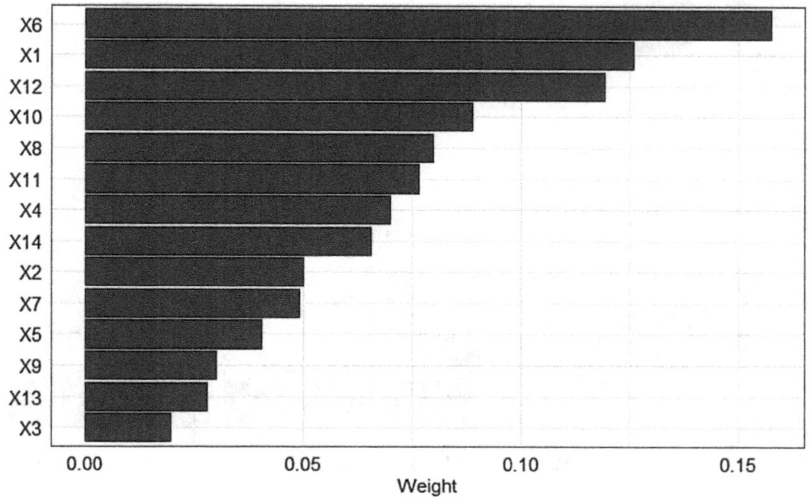

Fig. 4.2 WQS: estimated weights in the NHANES dataset

Attempting to estimate a WQS regression model with the negative directionality assumption on these data does not provide any result but only a warning that all bootstrap samples include positive estimates. This is reassuring as we know that data have been simulated based on mechanisms that only include null or positive effects. In this situation, the cumulative effect can be interpreted as a cumulative mixture effect. On the other hand, when exposures contribute to either positive or negative directions, the two estimates of the β_1 parameter (β_1^+ and β_1^-) should be presented and respectively interpreted as *cumulative effect of exposures operating in the positive direction*, and *cumulative effect of exposures operating in the negative direction*.

In more complex and likely more realistic settings, it is common to observe the same exposure as contributing to both the positive and negative indices. This is usually a sign that the relationship between that specific exposure and the outcome involves complex mechanisms that include non-linear and non-additive effects. In this situation the interpretation of the parameters can be revised into the cumulative effect of *mixture mechanisms* operating in the positive or negative direction.

4.3.3 Extensions of the WQS Framework

Repeated Holdout Validation for WQS Regression

One limitation of WQS is the reduced statistical power induced by splitting the dataset in training and validation sets. This partition can also lead to unrepresentative sets of data and unstable parameter estimates. An extension of the original

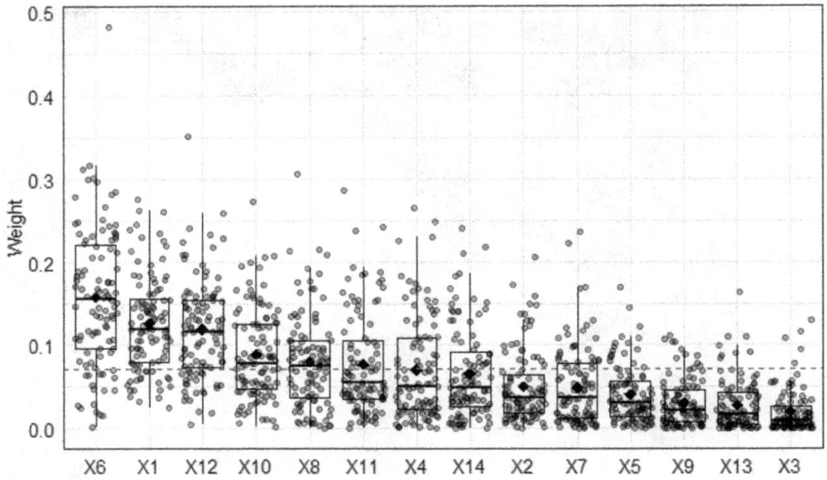

Fig. 4.3 WQS: estimated weights with repeated holdouts in the NHANES dataset

framework [52] showed that conducing a WQS regression on the full dataset without data splitting can produce optimistic results, and proposed to apply a repeated holdout validation combining cross-validation and bootstrap resampling. In practice, the data is randomly partitioned a k number of times, and a distribution of results in each validation set is produced. The authors recommend using $k = 100$ holdouts that, combined to the 100 bootstrap iterations in each resampling, might make the procedure computationally demanding in some situations. When a repeated holdout validation is chosen, a distribution of weights is obtained, allowing them to be presented with measures of variability across holdouts. For example, Fig. 4.3—produced by the `gwqs_barplot` function from the `gWQS` R package—includes a boxplot for each weight. The use of repeated holdouts allows incorporating measures of uncertainty for the weight estimation. Specifically, the dashed horizontal line in Fig. 4.3 is used to indicate *probable* contributors to the cumulative effect. The line is set at a level of $1/p$, where p is the number of exposures. A given exposure is considered a probable contributor to the overall mixture effect when it is above the threshold in at least 50% of the repeated holdouts (see Busgang et al. [4] for a detailed definition of this threshold computation).

Penalized Weights and Two Indices

A recent extension presented in Renzetti et al. [42] introduced a procedure where both a negative and a positive index can be estimated within the same statistical model. This approach includes a penalization term when estimating the weights and has the potential to improve estimation accuracy when the mixture components have both protective and harmful effects.

Zero-Inflated Exposures
The WQS regression can be generalized and applied to multiple types of dependent variables. In particular, WQS regression has been adapted to four different cases: logistic, multinomial, Poisson, and negative binomial regression. For the latter two cases, it is also possible to incorporate zero-inflated covariates. A standard Poisson and negative binomial objective function is used to estimate the weights, and zero inflation is accounted when fitting the model in the validation set.

Random Subset
WQS regression has been extended to deal with high-dimensional mixtures with highly correlated components [11]. This approach applies a random selection of a subset of the variables included in the mixture instead of the bootstrapping for parameter estimation. Through this method a more de-correlated subset of variables is generated, reducing the variance of the parameter estimates compared to a single analysis. This extension was shown to be more effective than WQS in modeling contexts with large predictor sets, complex correlation structures, or where the number of predictors exceeds the number of subjects.

Lagged WQS
Lagged WQS was introduced to incorporate time-varying effects in the mixture-health association and to understand the role of exposure timing in determining the health effects [17, 30]. This is an extension of high potential in the context of epidemiologic studies with repeated exposure measurements where the goal is to provide insights on the time-varying dimension of mixture effects.

Bayesian Weighted Indexes
Several papers have discussed weighted sum approaches within a Bayesian framework [10, 20, 55]. The approach proposed by Colicino et al. [10], in particular, directly extends the WQS framework (Bayesian WQS—BWQS) providing some additional levels of flexibility that can be useful in many settings. Several successful applications of BWQS have been presented in the literature (see, e.g., [6, 9, 34, 36]).

Permutation Test-Based Approach
A study by Day et al. [13] discussed permutation tests as an alternative way to data splitting and repeated holdout validation for assessing the significance of WQS results. The study observed optimal balance of power and false-positive rates when combining WQS with this permutation test. Of note, these results are based on simulations and, at the time of this writing, have not undergone substantial validation.

4.3.4 Quantile G-computation

Quantile G-computation was introduced by Keil et al. [24] as a novel statistical approach based on weighted indexing that attempts to strengthen the interpretation of findings from a causal inference perspective. This is achieved by integrating

WQS regression within G-computation, a powerful causal inference framework [33, 37]. Specifically, quantile G-computation follows a similar procedure as the one used by WQS but estimates the parameters of a marginal structural model rather than a GLM. In this way, under common assumptions in causal inference such as exchangeability, causal consistency, positivity, no interference, and correct model specification, this approach is expected to strongly increase the causal interpretation of the overall effect.[5] The modeling choice of quantile G-computation offers substantial advantages in terms of model flexibility. In particular, quantile G-computation does not make any unidirectionality assumption and allows incorporating non-linearities and non-additivities when defining the contribution of each exposure to the score. Of note, in addition to continuous, binary, and multinomial outcomes, the model can also be used to evaluate time-to-event data in the presence of right-censored survival outcomes. The approach is fully implemented in the R package `qgcomp`, which is accompanied by several comprehensive tutorials.

The flexibility of the approach comes with a price. In particular, the unconstrained nature of the weights (i.e., without directionality assumption) removes the main property that was preventing WQS results to be potentially affected by the reversal paradox. Application of quantile G-computation in the NHANES illustrative dataset, for example, suggests the presence of opposite effects for pairs of correlated predictors (Fig. 4.4), strongly resembling results from multivariable regression. In particular, the model indicates the presence of a contribution in the negative direction for X_3, highly correlated with X_4 and X_5, and for X_{13}, highly correlated with X_{12}, results that we know from simulations to be incorrect. Of note, however, this figure (which is here included as provided by default from the `plot` function in the `qgcomp` R package—version 2.15.2), can be misleading and should be interpreted with caution. Specifically, one might be led to conclude that X_3 and X_{13} are the two components providing the strongest contribution to the overall mixture effect. This, however, is simply due to the fact that both negative and positive weights have to sum up to 1. Therefore, the left and right side of the figure should not be compared to each other. The estimate of the overall mixture effect confirms that these negative weights do not substantially affect the overall effect. The estimate of β_1 when using quartiles for exposure categorizations is 0.29 (95% CI=0.21–0.36), remarkably similar to the one obtained by WQS.

Quantile G-computation integrates a direct estimation of the model parameters of the marginal structural model as well as an estimation procedure via bootstrap, both integrated in the R package. The approach has mostly received positive feedback [46] from the community and has already been successfully applied in a variety of contexts (see, e.g., [47, 51, 56]), also describing a Bayesian extension of the framework [23]. It is nevertheless important to remember that the weights estimation from quantile G-computation might be subject to potential bias in the presence of highly correlated exposures. In such settings, inference on the weights should be treated with caution.

---

[5] Issues around estimating causal effects in mixture analysis are further discussed in Sec. 6.1.

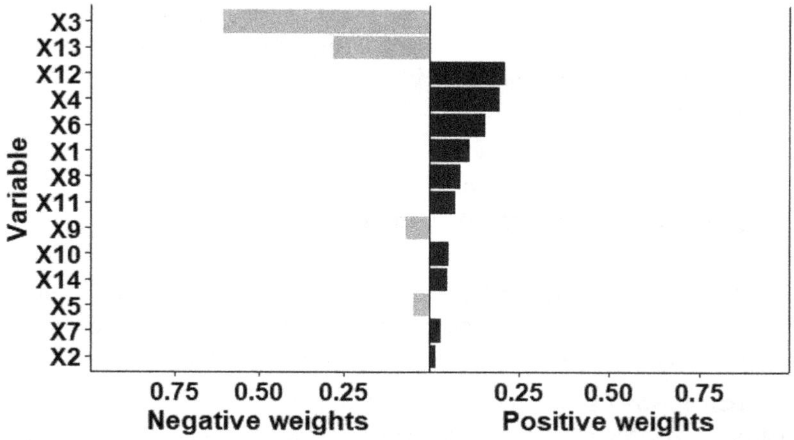

Fig. 4.4 Quantile G-computation: estimated weights in the NHANES dataset

4.3.5 WQS: Concluding Remarks

Indexing approaches provide unique features that allow for addressing two of the main research questions in the context of environmental mixtures analysis:

- What is the overall mixture effect?
- Who are the bad actors contributing to such effect?

WQS regression provides a robust procedure that is easy to implement and well documented. The hundreds of applications to date have proven the approach robust to several data structures and types of environmental exposures. Successful applications of the method have also been described in different fields outside of environmental epidemiology [19, 38]. The unidirectionality assumption prevents the appearance of noisy results due to the high levels of correlations, making WQS of particular appeal when the goal is to identify bad actors within a set of highly correlated predictors. The motivating examples behind the original development of WQS centered around toxicological questions on identifying bad actors in complex settings [12, 16]. To this extent, the assumption of unidirectionality was critical to disentangle the different mechanisms within the mixture operating in both directions [15]. At the same time, this assumption requires a cautious interpretation of the cumulative effect at the population level. Quantile G-computation, by relaxing this assumption of unidirectionality, allows a more robust estimation of the causal cumulative effects of exposure to the mixture at the population level. The difference in the goals and interpretation of the two approaches should be taken into account when deciding which approach should be used in a given context [15, 25].

In conclusion, the statistical framework of WQS and its extensions, including quantile G-computation, provides unique advantages and should be considered, together with regression modeling, as a key component of any analytical plan attempting to provide a comprehensive assessment of the health effects of mixture exposures. The choice of the specific approach within the framework should be selected on a case-by-case setting, and it is recommended to compare results under different modeling approaches.

4.4 Alternative Supervised Approaches

WQS and its extensions are not the only existing supervised indexing approaches. Alternative methods have been proposed and applied for the assessment of mixture-health associations and could be considered in specific settings.

Partial Least Square Regression
The Partial Least Square (PLS) regression can be thought of as a method that generalizes and combines PCA and multiple regression. PLS regression is very useful to predict dependent variables from a very large number of predictors that might be highly correlated. The PLS regression replaces the initial independent variable space (X) and the initial response variable space (Y) by smaller spaces that rely on a reduced number of variables named latent variables, which are included one by one in an iterative process. The sparse PLS (sPLS) regression, in particular, is an extension of PLS that aims at combining variable selection and modeling in a one-step procedure [27]. Components are defined iteratively such that they explain as much as possible of the remaining covariance between the predictors and the outcome. The sPLS approach simultaneously yields good predictive performance and appropriate variable selection by creating sparse linear combinations of the original predictors. Sparsity is induced by including a penalty in the estimation of the linear combination coefficients, that is, all coefficients with an absolute value lower than some fraction of the maximum absolute coefficient are shrunk to zero. sPLS is available in the R package `spls`. A detailed illustration of using sPLS in environmental epidemiology can be found in Lenters et al. [29].

Partial-Linear Single-Index Models
Partial-Linear Single-Index models are a family of semi-parametric models that attempt reducing a set of covariates to a single index within a regression framework [7]. This class of models can flexibly incorporate time-to-event outcomes [50] as well as longitudinal modeling [32], and has been proposed as a suitable approach that can handle some of the complexities of environmental mixtures [54].

Environmental Risk Scores
Another approach to incorporate several exposures into a single index is to apply the idea of risk modeling [49] to the analysis of environmental mixtures. This approach was originally proposed by Park et al. [39] based on aggregating multiple regression coefficients for selected mixture components. A later extension [40] has greatly improved the flexibility of this approach by incorporating a procedure where results from several different approaches for environmental mixtures are taken into

account for the selection of covariates included in the final environmental risk scores. Additional examples of environmental risk score modeling applications can be found in Balavarca et al. [2] and Pries et al. [41].

References

1. Peter C Austin. An introduction to propensity score methods for reducing the effects of confounding in observational studies. *Multivariate behavioral research*, 46(3):399–424, 2011.
2. Yesilda Balavarca, Korbinian Weigl, Hauke Thomsen, and Hermann Brenner. Performance of individual and joint risk stratification by an environmental risk score and a genetic risk score in a colorectal cancer screening setting. *International journal of cancer*, 146(3):627–634, 2020.
3. Kenneth A Bollen. Latent variables in psychology and the social sciences. *Annual review of psychology*, 53(1):605–634, 2002.
4. Stefanie A Busgang, Emily A Spear, Syam S Andra, Srinivasan Narasimhan, Jennifer B Bragg, Stefano Renzetti, Paul Curtin, Mia Bates, Manish Arora, Chris Gennings, et al. Application of growth modeling to assess the impact of hospital-based phthalate exposure on preterm infant growth parameters during the neonatal intensive care unit hospitalization. *Science of The Total Environment*, 850:157830, 2022.
5. Caroline Carrico, Chris Gennings, David C Wheeler, and Pam Factor-Litvak. Characterization of weighted quantile sum regression for highly correlated data in a risk analysis setting. *Journal of agricultural, biological, and environmental statistics*, 20(1):100–120, 2015.
6. Daniel Carrión, Elena Colicino, Nicolo Foppa Pedretti, Kodi B Arfer, Johnathan Rush, Nicholas DeFelice, and Allan C Just. Neighborhood-level disparities and subway utilization during the covid-19 pandemic in new york city. *Nature communications*, 12(1):3692, 2021.
7. Raymond J Carroll, Jianqing Fan, Irene Gijbels, and Matt P Wand. Generalized partially linear single-index models. *Journal of the American Statistical Association*, 92(438):477–489, 1997.
8. Krista Christensen, Jon Sobus, Martin Phillips, Todd Blessinger, Matthew Lorber, and Yu-Mei Tan. Changes in epidemiologic associations with different exposure metrics: a case study of phthalate exposure associations with body mass index and waist circumference. *Environment international*, 73:66–76, 2014.
9. Nathan J Cohen, Meizhen Yao, Vishal Midya, Sandra India-Aldana, Tomer Mouzica, Syam S Andra, Srinivasan Narasimhan, Anil K Meher, Manish Arora, Jerry Kok Yen Chan, et al. Exposure to perfluoroalkyl substances and women's fertility outcomes in a singaporean population-based preconception cohort. *Science of The Total Environment*, 873:162267, 2023.
10. Elena Colicino, Nicolo Foppa Pedretti, Stefanie A Busgang, and Chris Gennings. Per-and poly-fluoroalkyl substances and bone mineral density: Results from the bayesian weighted quantile sum regression. *Environmental Epidemiology (Philadelphia, Pa.)*, 4(3), 2020.
11. Paul Curtin, Joshua Kellogg, Nadja Cech, and Chris Gennings. A random subset implementation of weighted quantile sum (wqsrs) regression for analysis of high-dimensional mixtures. *Communications in Statistics-Simulation and Computation*, 50(4):1119–1134, 2021.
12. Jenna Czarnota, Chris Gennings, and David C Wheeler. Assessment of weighted quantile sum regression for modeling chemical mixtures and cancer risk. *Cancer informatics*, 14:CIN–S17295, 2015.
13. Drew B Day, Sheela Sathyanarayana, Kaja Z LeWinn, Catherine J Karr, W Alex Mason, and Adam A Szpiro. A permutation test-based approach to strengthening inference on the effects of environmental mixtures: comparison between single-index analytic methods. *Environmental health perspectives*, 130(8):087010, 2022.
14. Maya A Deyssenroth, Chris Gennings, Shelley H Liu, Shouneng Peng, Ke Hao, Luca Lambertini, Brian P Jackson, Margaret R Karagas, Carmen J Marsit, and Jia Chen. Intrauterine multi-metal exposure is associated with reduced fetal growth through modulation of the placental gene network. *Environment international*, 120:373–381, 2018.

15. Chris Gennings. Comment on 'a quantile-based g-computation approach to addressing the effects of exposure mixtures'. *Environmental health perspectives*, 129(3), 2021.
16. Chris Gennings, Caroline Carrico, Pam Factor-Litvak, Nickilou Krigbaum, Piera M Cirillo, and Barbara A Cohn. A cohort study evaluation of maternal pcb exposure related to time to pregnancy in daughters. *Environmental Health*, 12:1–12, 2013.
17. Chris Gennings, Paul Curtin, Ghalib Bello, Robert Wright, Manish Arora, and Christine Austin. Lagged wqs regression for mixtures with many components. *Environmental research*, 186:109529, 2020.
18. Alexios Ghalanos and Stefan Theussl. Rsolnp: general non-linear optimization using augmented lagrange multiplier method. *R package version*, 1, 2012.
19. Paul M Haller, Petr Jarolim, Michael G Palazzolo, Andrea Bellavia, Elliott M Antman, John Eikelboom, Christopher B Granger, Josephine Harrington, Jeff S Healey, Ziad Hijazi, et al. Heart failure risk assessment using biomarkers in patients with atrial fibrillation: analysis from combine-af. *Journal of the American College of Cardiology*, 2024.
20. Ghassan B Hamra, Richard F Maclehose, Lisa Croen, Elizabeth M Kauffman, and Craig Newschaffer. Bayesian weighted sums: a flexible approach to estimate summed mixture effects. *International journal of environmental research and public health*, 18(4):1373, 2021.
21. Russ Hauser and AM Calafat. Phthalates and human health. *Occupational and environmental medicine*, 62(11):806–818, 2005.
22. Tamarra James-Todd, Marta Ponzano, Andrea Bellavia, Paige L Williams, David E Cantonwine, Antonia M Calafat, Russ Hauser, Marlee R Quinn, Ellen W Seely, and Thomas F McElrath. Urinary phthalate and dinch metabolite concentrations and gradations of maternal glucose intolerance. *Environment international*, 161:107099, 2022.
23. Alexander P Keil, Jessie P Buckley, and Amy E Kalkbrenner. Bayesian g-computation for estimating impacts of interventions on exposure mixtures: demonstration with metals from coal-fired power plants and birth weight. *American journal of epidemiology*, 190(12):2647–2657, 2021.
24. Alexander P Keil, Jessie P Buckley, Katie M O'Brien, Kelly K Ferguson, Shanshan Zhao, and Alexandra J White. A quantile-based g-computation approach to addressing the effects of exposure mixtures. *Environmental health perspectives*, 128(4):047004, 2020.
25. Alexander P Keil, Jessie P Buckley, Katie M O'brien, Kelly K Ferguson, Shanshan Zhao, and Alexandra J White. Response to "comment on 'a quantile-based g-computation approach to addressing the effects of exposure mixtures'". *Environmental health perspectives*, 129(3):038002, 2021.
26. Holger M Koch, Bernd Rossbach, Hans Drexler, and Jürgen Angerer. Internal exposure of the general population to dehp and other phthalates—determination of secondary and primary phthalate monoester metabolites in urine. *Environmental research*, 93(2):177–185, 2003.
27. Kim-Anh Lê Cao, Debra Rossouw, Christele Robert-Granié, and Philippe Besse. A sparse pls for variable selection when integrating omics data. *Statistical applications in genetics and molecular biology*, 7(1), 2008.
28. Wan-Chen Lee, Mandy Fisher, Karelyn Davis, Tye E Arbuckle, and Sanjoy K Sinha. Identification of chemical mixtures to which canadian pregnant women are exposed: The mirec study. *Environment international*, 99:321–330, 2017.
29. Virissa Lenters, Lützen Portengen, Lidwien AM Smit, Bo AG Jönsson, Aleksander Giwercman, Lars Rylander, Christian H Lindh, Marcello Spanò, Henning S Pedersen, Jan K Ludwicki, et al. Phthalates, perfluoroalkyl acids, metals and organochlorines and reproductive function: a multipollutant assessment in greenlandic, polish and ukrainian men. *Occupational and environmental medicine*, 72(6):385–393, 2015.
30. Yuri Levin-Schwartz, Chris Gennings, Lourdes Schnaas, María del Carmen Hernández Chávez, David C Bellinger, Martha Maria Téllez-Rojo, Andrea A Baccarelli, and Robert O Wright. Time-varying associations between prenatal metal mixtures and rapid visual processing in children. *Environmental Health*, 18:1–12, 2019.
31. Cathryn M Lewis and Evangelos Vassos. Polygenic risk scores: from research tools to clinical instruments. *Genome medicine*, 12(1):44, 2020.

32. Gaorong Li, Lixing Zhu, Liugen Xue, and Sanying Feng. Empirical likelihood inference in partially linear single-index models for longitudinal data. *Journal of Multivariate Analysis*, 101(3):718–732, 2010.
33. Sean McGrath, Victoria Lin, Zilu Zhang, Lucia C Petito, Roger W Logan, Miguel A Hernán, and Jessica G Young. gformula: an r package for estimating the effects of sustained treatment strategies via the parametric g-formula. *Patterns*, 1(3), 2020.
34. Vishal Midya, Elena Colicino, David V Conti, Kiros Berhane, Erika Garcia, Nikos Stratakis, Sandra Andrusaityte, Xavier Basagaña, Maribel Casas, Serena Fossati, et al. Association of prenatal exposure to endocrine-disrupting chemicals with liver injury in children. *JAMA Network Open*, 5(7):e2220176–e2220176, 2022.
35. Lidia Mínguez-Alarcón, Carmen Messerlian, Andrea Bellavia, Audrey J Gaskins, Yu-Han Chiu, Jennifer B Ford, Alexandra R Azevedo, John C Petrozza, Antonia M Calafat, Russ Hauser, et al. Urinary concentrations of bisphenol a, parabens and phthalate metabolite mixtures in relation to reproductive success among women undergoing in vitro fertilization. *Environment international*, 126:355–362, 2019.
36. Vicente Mustieles, Matthieu Rolland, Isabelle Pin, Cathrine Thomsen, Amrit K Sakhi, Azemira Sabaredzovic, Gina Muckle, Karine Guichardet, Rémy Slama, and Claire Philippat. Early-life exposure to a mixture of phenols and phthalates in relation to child social behavior: applying an evidence-based prioritization to a cohort with improved exposure assessment. *Environmental Health Perspectives*, 131(8):087006, 2023.
37. Ashley I Naimi, Stephen R Cole, and Edward H Kennedy. An introduction to g methods. *International journal of epidemiology*, 46(2):756–762, 2017.
38. Jeri W Nieves, Chris Gennings, Pam Factor-Litvak, Jonathan Hupf, Jessica Singleton, Valerie Sharf, Björn Oskarsson, J Americo M Fernandes Filho, Eric J Sorenson, Emanuele D'Amico, et al. Association between dietary intake and function in amyotrophic lateral sclerosis. *JAMA neurology*, 73(12):1425–1432, 2016.
39. Sung Kyun Park, Yebin Tao, John D Meeker, Siobán D Harlow, and Bhramar Mukherjee. Environmental risk score as a new tool to examine multi-pollutants in epidemiologic research: an example from the nhanes study using serum lipid levels. *PloS one*, 9(6):e98632, 2014.
40. Sung Kyun Park, Zhangchen Zhao, and Bhramar Mukherjee. Construction of environmental risk score beyond standard linear models using machine learning methods: application to metal mixtures, oxidative stress and cardiovascular disease in nhanes. *Environmental Health*, 16:1–17, 2017.
41. Lotta-Katrin Pries, Gamze Erzin, Bart PF Rutten, Jim van Os, and Sinan Guloksuz. Estimating aggregate environmental risk score in psychiatry: the exposome score for schizophrenia. *Frontiers in psychiatry*, 12:671334, 2021.
42. Stefano Renzetti, Chris Gennings, and Stefano Calza. A weighted quantile sum regression with penalized weights and two indices. *Frontiers in Public Health*, 11:1151821, 2023.
43. Guillaume Rousselet, Cyril R Pernet, and Rand R Wilcox. An introduction to the bootstrap: a versatile method to make inferences by using data-driven simulations. *Meta-Psychology*, 7, 2023.
44. Amrit Kaur Sakhi, Azemira Sabaredzovic, Enrique Cequier, and Cathrine Thomsen. Phthalate metabolites in norwegian mothers and children: Levels, diurnal variation and use of personal care products. *Science of the Total Environment*, 599:1984–1992, 2017.
45. Tiffany R Sanchez, Vesna Slavkovich, Nancy LoIacono, Alexander van Geen, Tyler Ellis, Steven N Chillrud, Olgica Balac, Tarique Islam, Faruque Parvez, Habib Ahsan, et al. Urinary metals and metal mixtures in bangladesh: exploring environmental sources in the health effects of arsenic longitudinal study (heals). *Environment international*, 121:852–860, 2018.
46. Silke Schmidt. Quantile g-computation: a new method for analyzing mixtures of environmental exposures. *Environmental health perspectives*, 128(10):104004, 2020.
47. Thea S Skogheim, Kjell Vegard F Weyde, Stephanie M Engel, Heidi Aase, Pål Surén, Merete G Øie, Guido Biele, Ted Reichborn-Kjennerud, Ida H Caspersen, Mady Hornig, et al. Metal and essential element concentrations during pregnancy and associations with autism spectrum

disorder and attention-deficit/hyperactivity disorder in children. *Environment international*, 152:106468, 2021.
48. Irene Souter, Andrea Bellavia, Paige L Williams, TIM Korevaar, John D Meeker, Joseph M Braun, Ralph A de Poortere, Maarten A Broeren, Jennifer B Ford, Antonia M Calafat, et al. Urinary concentrations of phthalate metabolite mixtures in relation to serum biomarkers of thyroid function and autoimmunity among women from a fertility center. *Environmental health perspectives*, 128(6):067007, 2020.
49. Ewout W Steyerberg and Ewout W Steyerberg. Applications of prediction models. *Clinical prediction models: a practical approach to development, validation, and updating*, pages 15–36, 2019.
50. Jie Sun, Karen A Kopciuk, and Xuewen Lu. Polynomial spline estimation of partially linear single-index proportional hazards regression models. *Computational statistics & data analysis*, 53(1):176–188, 2008.
51. Yi Sun, Xia Li, Tarik Benmarhnia, Jiu-Chiuan Chen, Chantal Avila, David A Sacks, Vicki Chiu, Jeff Slezak, John Molitor, Darios Getahun, et al. Exposure to air pollutant mixture and gestational diabetes mellitus in southern california: Results from electronic health record data of a large pregnancy cohort. *Environment international*, 158:106888, 2022.
52. Eva M Tanner, Carl-Gustaf Bornehag, and Chris Gennings. Repeated holdout validation for weighted quantile sum regression. *MethodsX*, 6:2855–2860, 2019.
53. Hexing Wang, Ying Zhou, Chuanxi Tang, Yanhong He, Jingui Wu, Yue Chen, and Qingwu Jiang. Urinary phthalate metabolites are associated with body mass index and waist circumference in chinese school children. *PloS one*, 8(2):e56800, 2013.
54. Yuyan Wang, Yinxiang Wu, Melanie H Jacobson, Myeonggyun Lee, Peng Jin, Leonardo Trasande, and Mengling Liu. A family of partial-linear single-index models for analyzing complex environmental exposures with continuous, categorical, time-to-event, and longitudinal health outcomes. *Environmental Health*, 19:1–16, 2020.
55. David C Wheeler, Salem Rustom, Matthew Carli, Todd P Whitehead, Mary H Ward, and Catherine Metayer. Bayesian group index regression for modeling chemical mixtures and cancer risk. *International Journal of Environmental Research and Public Health*, 18(7):3486, 2021.
56. Jie Zhang, Xin-Yu Fang, Jun Wu, Yin-Guang Fan, Rui-Xue Leng, Bo Liu, Xiao-Jie Lv, Yu-Lu Yan, Chen Mao, and Dong-Qing Ye. Association of combined exposure to ambient air pollutants, genetic risk, and incident rheumatoid arthritis: a prospective cohort study in the uk biobank. *Environmental Health Perspectives*, 131(3):037008, 2023.

Chapter 5
Flexible Approaches for Complex Settings

5.1 Assumptions of Linearity and Additivity in Regression Modeling

The previous chapters of this book described the use of regression-based approaches for environmental mixtures. Whether directly focusing on mixture components (Chap. 3) or on a summary score of the mixture (Chap. 4), the statistical methods we have described are all grounded within the familiar setting of regression modeling and its extensions. The flexibility of regression approaches and its advantages in terms of results interpretation rely on whether the assumptions made by the chosen model are met in the data. There are two important assumptions that require extensive attention in the context of environmental mixtures: linearity and additivity. These assumptions are implicitly made by all the most common regression approaches used in clinical and epidemiologic research, including GLM (linear, logistic, and Poisson regression), Cox regression models, accelerated failure times models, and many others. Assumptions of linearity are made for each continuous covariate included in the model, while assumptions of additivity are made for each combination of covariates, regardless of their nature. Therefore, when incorporating multiple environmental exposures in the same regression model, we are implicitly making a substantial number of assumptions that should be carefully evaluated and potentially addressed. The next subsection provides a more formal introduction to the concepts of linearity and additivity in regression modeling, discussing available tools to relax these assumptions and challenges with implementing them in the context of environmental mixtures, and introduces the notion of model overfitting. The following sections will then introduce two flexible statistical frameworks for environmental mixtures that can account for non-linear and non-additive effects: Bayesian Kernel Machine Regression (BKMR) and Generalized Additive Models (GAMs). Finally, the last section of this chapter will provide a general introduction to the application of machine learning (ML) for environmental mixtures research,

A. Bellavia, *Statistical Methods for Environmental Mixtures*, Society, Environment and Statistics, https://doi.org/10.1007/978-3-031-78987-8_5

discussing the settings where these could provide advantages and the challenges involved in their application.

Let's begin from a simple setting with a continuous outcome Y and two environmental factors X_1 and X_2. We can assume for simplicity that the two factors are not highly correlated, and we can fit a multivariable model without any risk of collinearity:

$$Y_i = \beta_0 + \beta_1 \cdot X_{1i} + \beta_2 \cdot X_{2i} + \epsilon_i \quad (5.1)$$

In addition to the standard assumptions of a linear regression model (normality and homoscedasticity), Eq. 5.1 assumes:

- Linearity in the association between both X_1 and X_2 and the outcome Y
- Additivity of the effects of the two variables

5.1.1 Relaxing Linearity

Assumptions of linearity are made for each continuous covariate in the model. For example, one of the assumptions of the regression model from Eq. 5.1 is that the effect of X_1 on Y will be the same for each unit increase in the exposure. As an illustrative example, imagine we want to study the relationship between a continuous exposure X_1 and a continuous outcome Y. The data points presented in Fig. 5.1 show the real relationship between X_1 and Y, displaying a U-shape. The linearity assumption that a linear regression model would implicitly make is described by the dotted line, showing the model fit of such regression. To relax this unrealistic assumption and improve model fitting, a common alternative is to consider a categorical transformation of the continuous predictor, dividing for example its distribution into quartiles. Results from this approach would provide the fit described by the dashed line in Fig. 5.1. Categorizing continuous predictors, however, only replaces the linearity assumption with the alternative assumption that the functional form relating exposure and outcome is a step function. Limitations of this categorical approach have been long recognized [31, 80], and alternative options have been suggested [32, 34, 81]. Among these, a recommended solution is to use smoothed nonparametric estimation based on *spline transformations* [38]. Spline transformations relax any assumptions on the functional form relating exposures and outcome and rather let the data suggest the shape of the exposure-response relationship. This is generally achieved by selecting specific points of the exposure distribution, referred to as *knots* (e.g., the 10th, 50th, and 90th percentiles of the distribution) and by using cubic polynomials to model the effect within knots. Even in the most simplified settings, a spline transformation for a single covariate requires the inclusion of at least two regression coefficients, thus increasing the number of parameters to be estimated and the complexity of the model [38]. The result of this increased complexity, nevertheless, is a considerable improvement in model fitting, as intuitively shown by the solid curve in Fig. 5.1.

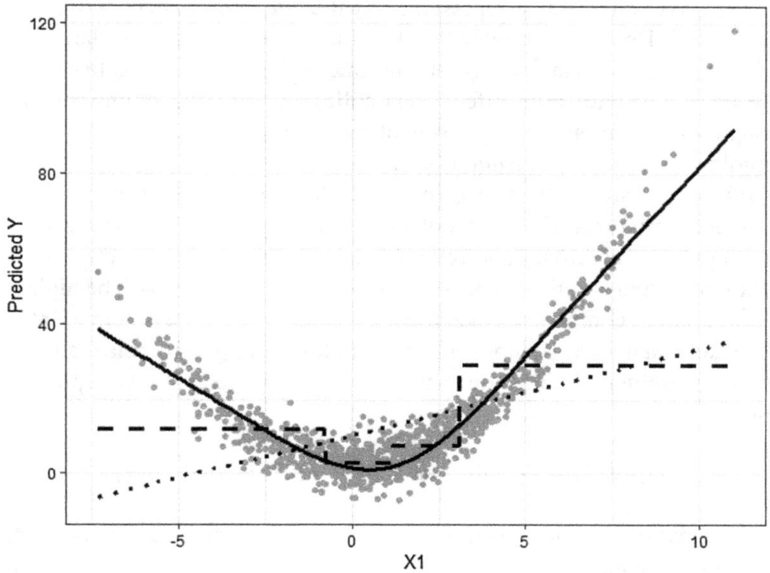

Fig. 5.1 Model fit from linear (dotted line), categorical (dashed line), and spline transformation (solid line)

5.1.2 Relaxing Additivity

The assumption of additivity relates to the way the different covariates in a regression model affect each other in predicting the outcome. Specifically, a regression model as defined in Eq. 5.1 assumes that the individual estimates of each covariate (β_1 and β_2) are constant over levels of all the other covariates in the model. For example, $\hat{\beta}_1$ will represent the effect of increasing X_1 by one SD unit for any level of X_2, assuming all covariates have been standardized. This is translated into a specific assumption on the way the two covariates jointly operate. The implicit hypothesis of Eq. 5.1 is that the joint effect of the two exposures coincides to the sum of the two main effects ($\hat{\beta}_1 + \hat{\beta}_2$). Say, for example, that a SD-unit increase in pollutant 1 is expected to increase systolic blood pressure (SBP) by 1 mmHg, and a SD-unit increase in pollutant 2 will instead increase SBP by 2 mmHg. A regression model that includes both pollutants will make the implicit assumption that the increase in SBP when both factors jointly change by a SD-unit increase will be of 3 mmHg $(1 + 2)$.

This perfect additivity might be expected if the two factors of interest are operating through independent biological pathways. When focusing on environmental mixtures, however, there are several settings where this might not be the case [24, 44, 65, 89]. Two compounds of the same chemical class, for example, might share biological pathways and result in either a dilution of the joint effect (i.e., less than the sum) or an enhancement (i.e., more than the sum). The difference from the sum of the two main effects is represented by the *interaction* effect between the two covariates [94]. Depending on whether the joint effect is smaller or larger than the sum of the two main effects, we refer to this interaction as either negative or positive. The presence of an interaction effect also implies that the effect of one covariate will be stronger or weaker at varying levels of the other covariate, a concept known in epidemiology as *effect modification* [93].

To fully understand the processes through which components of a certain environmental mixtures affect the outcome, it is required to assess the validity of any assumption of additivity and relax these assumptions if not met in the data. It goes without saying that the chances of non-additive behaviors will be higher as the number of mixture components increases, thus making the assessment of interaction effects a key analytical component in complex settings. To relax additivity in regression modeling, we include a product term between the two predictors of interest:

$$Y_i = \beta_0 + \beta_1 \cdot X_{1i} + \beta_2 \cdot X_{2i} + \beta_3 \cdot X_{1i} \cdot X_{2i} + \epsilon_i \tag{5.2}$$

The estimate of β_3 from this model represents the interaction effect. If $\beta_3 = 0$, there is no interaction, and the joint effect corresponds to the sum of the two main effects (perfect additivity). If β_3 is either <0 or >0, we are instead in the presence of negative or positive interaction, respectively. Note that a negative interaction does not imply a negative joint effect. For example, using the previous example of how two pollutants affect SBP, a negative interaction of -0.5 would imply that the increase in SBP when both exposures jointly increase by one SD unit is 2.5 mmHg $(2 + 1 - 0.5)$.

5.1.3 *Model Overfitting*

As the number of mixture components increases, so does the number of assumptions that need to be assessed and potentially relaxed. Even in a simple setting with only three exposures (A, B, C), there are three potential splines transformations (at least six parameters) and three possible sets of two-way interactions (AxB, AxC, BxC) that could be explored. Higher-order interactions could also be considered as the number of exposures increases. For example, we might include a three-way interaction that describes how the joint effect of the three exposures differs from the sum of each main effect and each pair of two-way interactions. Relaxing all these assumptions through regression modeling is generally unfeasible as the number of parameters to be estimated increases drastically. In addition to computational and mathematical complexities, moreover, inclusion of non-linear and non-additive effects will increase the risk of *model overfitting*. Overfitting is a concept that describes those situations where the chosen analytical tool perfectly fits the data at the expense of poor generalizability in the external population [99]. When dealing with complex data, it is not always the case that complex models should be preferred. The question should rather be on what is the best model that can flexibly incorporate the required amount of complexity with limited loss in terms of generalizability [70]. In the next sections, we will describe alternative analytical approaches that can be considered in those settings where the data complexity makes regression of little use and at high risk of overfitting. All these approaches are able to flexibly incorporate complex non-linear and non-additive settings and target the problem of overfitting from different perspectives: Bayesian Kernel Machine Regression (Sect. 5.2) includes variable selection through a Bayesian procedure; generalized additive model (Sect. 5.3) include parameters penalization and variable selection; ML approaches (Sect. 5.4) use cross-validation.

5.2 Bayesian Kernel Machine Regression (BKMR)

5.2.1 Introduction

BKMR was first presented in Bobb et al. [13] as a flexible nonparametric approach that can target several objectives of mixtures research, including the detection and estimation of an effect of the overall mixture, identification of exposure or group of exposures responsible for observed mixture effects, visualizing the exposure-response function, and detection of interactions among individual exposures.

The foundation of BKMR is to model the environmental mixture through means of a kernel function. Kernel estimation is a powerful analytical tool for estimating multivariable predictor-outcome associations without explicit assumptions, while still adjusting for potential confounders. Specifically, the general modeling framework of BKMR is

$$Y_i = h(X_{i1}, \ldots, X_{iP}) + \beta c_i + \epsilon_i \tag{5.3}$$

where Y_i is a continuous, normally distributed health endpoint, h is a flexible function of the predictor variables $X_{i1}, \ldots, X_{iP}$ (the kernel function), and c_i is a vector of covariates assumed to have a linear relationship with the outcome.

There are several possible choices for the kernel function used to represent h. BKMR uses a Gaussian kernel, which flexibly captures a wide range of underlying functional forms for h and can accommodate non-linear and non-additive effects of the multivariate exposure. Specifically, an augmented Gaussian kernel is used, implying the following representation for h:

$$K_{vs}(X_i, X_j) = exp\{-\sum_P r_p(X_{ip} - X_{jp})^2\} \tag{5.4}$$

Intuitively, the kernel function shrinks the estimated health effects of two individuals with similar exposure profiles toward each other. The weights r_p are auxiliary variables of the augmented estimation that represent the probability that each exposure is important in the function, with $r_p = 0$ indicating that there is no association between the pth exposure and the outcome. By allowing some weights to be 0, the method is implicitly embedding a variable selection procedure—another useful property of kernel estimation [59, 84].

5.2.2 *Estimation*

Out of several potential approaches for kernel methods estimation, BKMR chooses a Bayesian approach.[1] Specifically, the model is fit using a hybrid Gibbs/Metropolis-Hastings Markov Chain Monte Carlo (MCMC), thoroughly described in Bobb et al. [13]. This approach requires providing prior distributions for all model parameters, including the auxiliary parameters r_p. The posterior estimates of these parameters will indicate the relative importance of each mixture component.

As common with iterative procedures based on MCMC, the interpretation of the results will strongly rely on whether parameters converge over the iterations. A simple tool to assess model convergence is provided by the *trace plots*. Figure 5.2 provides an example of a trace plot for one of the model parameters after applying BKMR with 1000 MCMC iterations in the NHANES data. As clearly visible from the figure, it takes the model about 100 iterations to converge to the final parameter estimate. These figures are not only necessary to check parameter convergence but also critical for removing the so-called burning phase. Final estimates will be calculated as an average over iterations, and it is, as such, important to remove the noise of early iterations. In this example we might consider removing the first 100 iterations. This would allow the final estimates to be calculated as an average of only the stable iterations, presented in Fig. 5.3.

5.2.3 *Variable Selection Procedures*

The iterative nature of MCMC allows describing variable importance in terms of Posterior Inclusion Probability (PIP), the proportion of iterations with $r_p > 0$. Typically, several thousands of iterations are required for a robust estimation of these probabilities. PIPs are estimated for each mixture component, thus providing a tool for *component-wise* variable selection. Components with a PIP of 0 are not selected and not considered for the final estimation of $h()$. As an important practical note, PIPs are continuous measures between 0 and 1 and should be interpreted in terms of relative importance of each component as compared to each other. There

[1] For a general introduction to Bayesian statistics for epidemiologists, including some core concepts used by BKMR such as MCMC and iterations, the reader can refer to this series of introductory papers by S. Greenland [33, 35, 36].

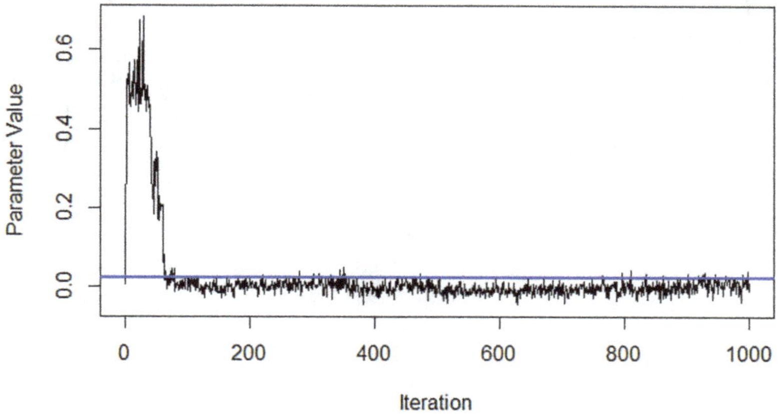

Fig. 5.2 BKMR: convergence plot for a single parameter

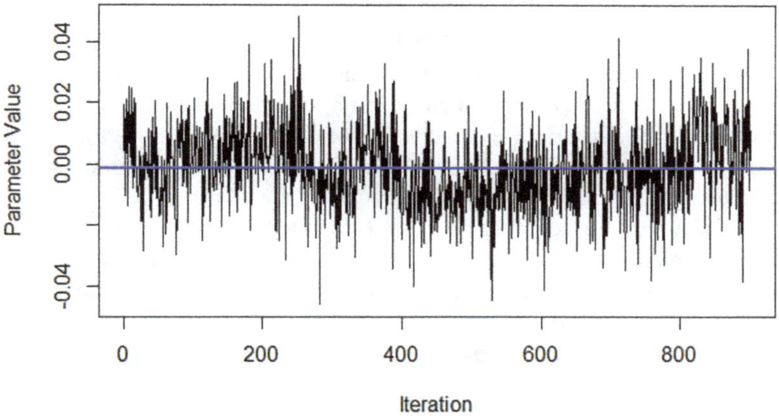

Fig. 5.3 BKMR: convergence plot for a single parameter after burning phase exclusion

are no thresholds of PIP that can be used to formally classify a specific mixture component as important vs non-important.

Table 5.1 shows PIPs estimated by BKMR with component-wise selection in the illustrative NHANES dataset. In descending order, the most important contribution seems to come from X_{12}, X_{10}, X_8, X_{11}, X_{14}, X_6.

A common problem with component-wise selection is that it is challenging to identify important variables within highly correlated groups of exposures. For example, Table 5.1 provides limited information on what components of the highly correlated $X_3 - X_5$ cluster, if any, are associated with the outcome. An alternative *hierarchical* selection has been developed to take into account structural properties of the mixture, such as its correlation. When this approach is chosen, PIPs are

Table 5.1 BKMR: Posterior Inclusion Probabilities in the NHANES dataset

	PIP
X_1	0.110
X_2	0.082
X_3	0
X_4	0
X_5	0.072
X_6	0.142
X_7	0
X_8	0.336
X_9	0.062
X_{10}	0.400
X_{11}	0.188
X_{12}	0.818
X_{13}	0.080
X_{14}	0.158

estimated at two levels: group-level PIPs, indicating the relative importance of a specific cluster, and individual-level PIPs, indicating the relative importance of each component within each cluster. When operating hierarchical selection, the specification of potential clusters of exposures is not data-driven but a priori defined by the user. As such, careful consideration should be made when defining subgroups, possibly using quantitative tools in support of the clustering (e.g., correlation structure, PCA results), together with prior knowledge on the biological structure of the environmental exposures. Ideally, exposures within the same subgroup in the hierarchical model should be expected to affect the outcome in the same direction and without interaction effects.

Using the NHANES dataset example, we could for instance inform the model that there are highly correlated clusters of exposures. This alternative modeling might provide additional insights on the relative importance of each cluster and of each exposure within it. Table 5.2, for example, provides PIP estimates from a BKMR with hierarchical selection where predictors were separated into two groups: the cluster of highly correlated covariates $X_3 - X_5$ (group 2) and all other covariates (group 1). Group PIPs indicate that the cluster is possibly relevant in the exposure-response association, while individual PIPs suggest that X_4 might be the most important of the three exposures. We know from the simulations that X_4 is indeed the only covariate of the highly correlated cluster to be really associated with the outcome. This was missed by the component-wise approach but is instead captured by the hierarchical selection. Nevertheless, positive PIPs are still estimated for the other member of the correlated clusters (X_3 and X_5) that, in reality, are not associated with the outcome.

Table 5.2 BKMR: Posterior Inclusion Probabilities from hierarchical BKMR in the simulated dataset

	Group	Group PIP	Individual PIP
X_1	1	1	0
X_2	1	1	0
X_3	2	0.044	0.364
X_4	2	0.044	0.455
X_5	2	0.044	0.182
X_6	1	1	0.016
X_7	1	1	0.004
X_8	1	1	0.062
X_9	1	1	0.054
X_{10}	1	1	0
X_{11}	1	1	0.002
X_{12}	1	1	0.450
X_{13}	1	1	0.146
X_{14}	1	1	0.266

5.2.4 Exposure-Outcome Function Characterization

The goal of BKMR is to flexibly estimate the association between several environmental factors and the outcome accounting for non-linear and non-additive effects. In such complex settings, it is not possible to provide a single comprehensive representation of the association. The model provides an estimate of the multidimensional function $h()$, and graphical tools should then be used to cross-section this function from specific dimensions of interest. There are several graphical tools that can be investigated for a comprehensive summary of results, all implemented in available software [12].

Univariate Exposure-Response Functions
A key cross section of interest is the univariate relationship between each covariate and the outcome, where all of the other exposures are fixed to a particular percentile, commonly their median. Figure 5.4 shows this result for the 14 NHANES dataset exposures, indicating that all selected covariates have weak to moderate associations with the outcome.[2]

Single Variable Effects
An alternative way to summarize individual effects is by looking at the contribution of an individual predictor to the response. For example, we may wish to compare the outcome when a single predictor in h is set at different percentiles of its distribution (e.g., 25th, 50th, 75th), setting all of the remaining predictors at a specific percentile (Fig. 5.5).

[2] Note the direct relationship between these results and PIP estimates reported in Table 5.1: exposures with PIP=0 (X_3, X_4, X_7) do not contribute to the estimation of $h()$ as documented by the straight horizontal line in this figure.

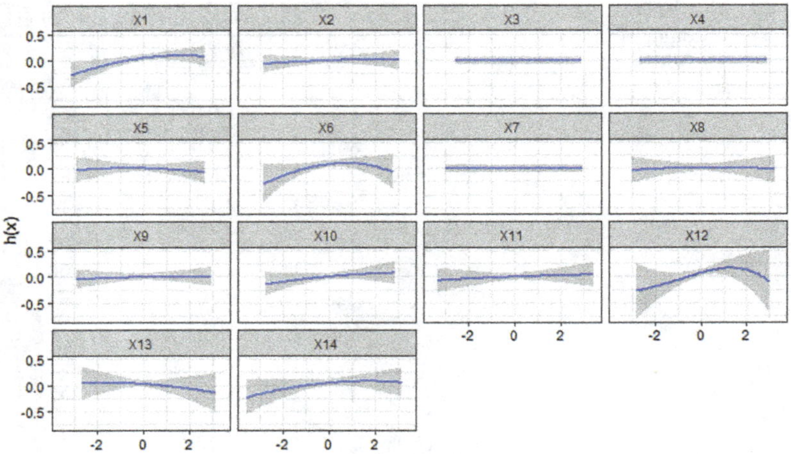

Fig. 5.4 BKMR: univariate exposure-response associations in the NHANES dataset

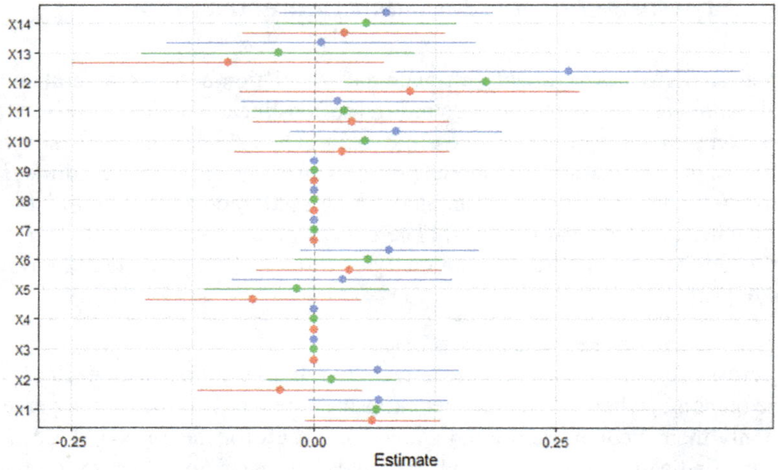

Fig. 5.5 BKMR: estimates of h function by fixing individual exposures at their 25th (red), 50th (green), and 75th (blue) percentiles

Bivariate Exposure-Response Functions

It is then useful to visualize the bivariate exposure-response function for two predictors, where all of the other predictors are fixed at a particular percentile, commonly the median. Visualizing each pair of exposures is non-straightforward, and it is recommended to only select relevant pairs of predictors, for example, focusing on two exposures for which a positive association has been observed at

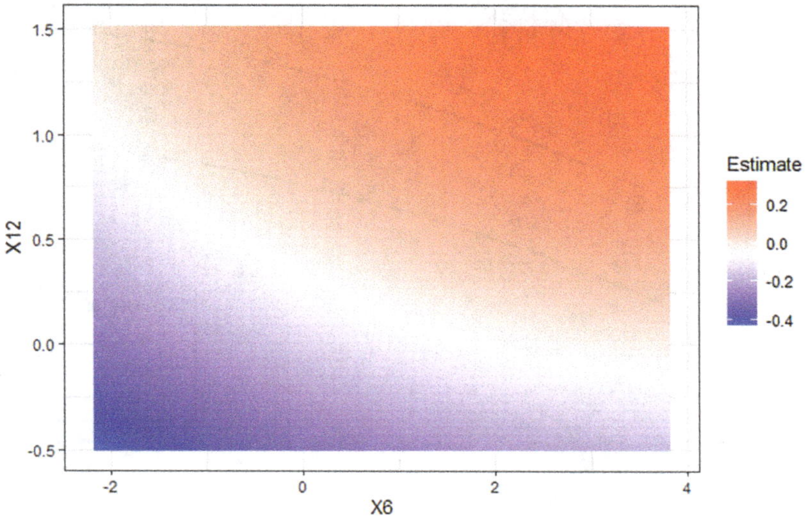

Fig. 5.6 BKMR: bivariate exposure-response association for joint levels of X_6 and X_{12} in the NHANES dataset

the univariate level. Figure 5.6, for example, presents this bivariate association for X_6 and X_{12}.[3]

Interactions

As described in 5.1.2, interactions between predictors would imply that the effect of a certain exposure varies over levels of the other exposure with which it interacts. An intuitive way of visualizing this behavior is to investigate the predictor-response function of a single predictor in X for a given second predictor in X fixed at various precentiles (and for the remaining predictors fixed to a specific value, commonly their median). This can be presented either for all possible combinations of predictors or for a selected pair of interest. Figure 5.7 shows the plot for the effect of X_6 on Y over levels of X_{12} in the NHANES data. The curves have the same shape, implying a possible absence of interactions.[4]

Interactions can also be summarized in terms of how much each predictor interacts with all other components of the mixtures. This can be achieved by displaying how the individual effects change when all of the other predictors in X are fixed to their 75th percentile to when all of the other predictors in X are fixed

[3] These bivariate plots, sometimes referred to as *contour plots*, are not of easy interpretation. It might be useful to think of them as hiking maps where the gradation in color indicates a change in elevation as a function of moving across latitude and longitude (i.e., the value of h as it changes moving in the space of the two covariates).

[4] This conclusion is correct. We know from simulations that there are no interactions between any pair of predictors.

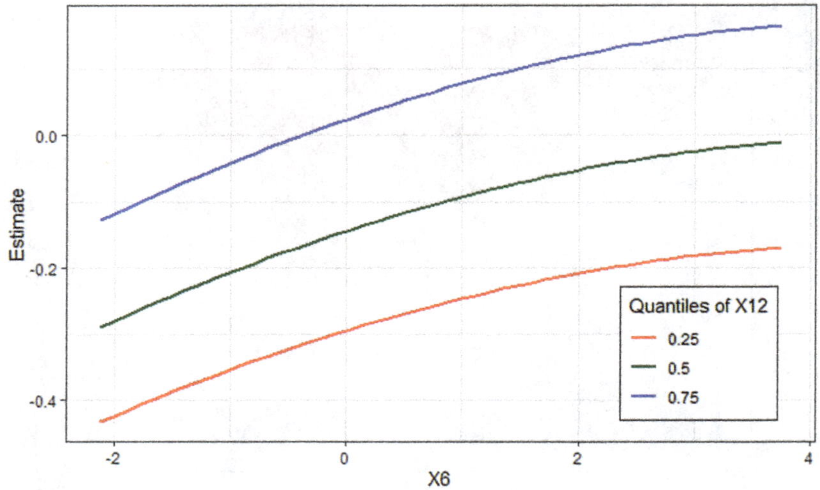

Fig. 5.7 BKMR: exposure-response association for X_6 at varying levels of X_{12} in the NHANES dataset

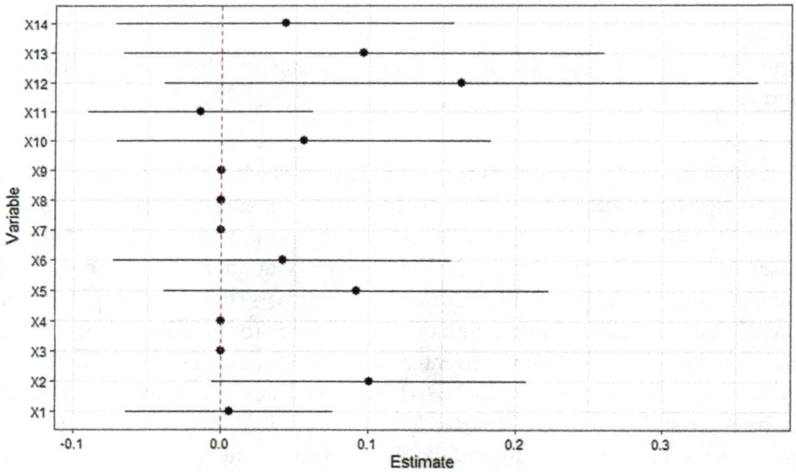

Fig. 5.8 BKMR: individual interaction effects in the NHANES dataset

to their 25th percentile (Fig. 5.8). As with the previous figure, this graph also leads us to conclude that we have no substantial evidence of interaction in this data.

Overall Mixture Effect

Finally, BKMR allows estimating a cumulative overall effect of the mixture, calculated by comparing the value of h when all predictors are set to a particular percentile as compared to when all of them are set to their 50th percentile (Fig. 5.9).

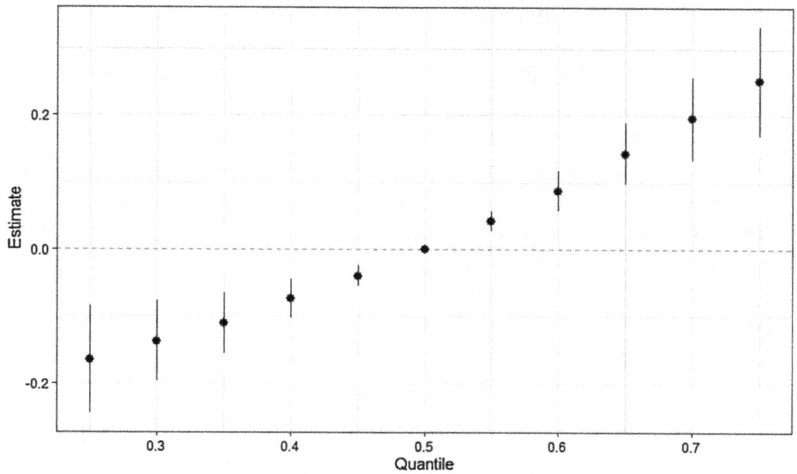

Fig. 5.9 BKMR: overall mixture effect in the NHANES dataset

In agreement with results from WQS and quantile G-computation, higher exposure to the overall mixture is associated with higher expected value of the outcome. Of note, as for all other plots presented, this is only calculated based on the exposures that were selected for the estimation of $h()$. As such, this figure is technically representing the cumulative effect of selected predictors, thus possibly underestimating the overall mixture effect.

5.2.5 Notes on Software Implementation

BKMR is fully implemented in the `bkmr` R package, developed by the authors and comprehensively presented in Bobb et al. [12]. In brief, the main functions of the package include:

- `kmbayes()` to fit the model through MCMC
- `tracePlots()` to visualize and study convergence and inform on burning phase removal
- `ExtractPIPs()` to display PIPs
- Functions to derive the presented plots:
  - `PredictorResponseUnivar()`
  - `PredictorResponseBivarLevels()`
  - `OverallRiskSummaries()`
  - `SingVarRiskSummaries()`
  - `SingVarIntSummaries()`

A couple of additional practical caveats are noteworthy. First, because of the iterative MCMC procedure implemented in the estimation, it is important to include a *seed* option for reproducible results. Second, especially with large datasets, the estimation becomes computationally intensive and might take hours to run. As an attempt to address this limitation, the authors have introduced an option to incorporate Gaussian predictive process [4] where a set of *knots* are selected over the exposure space and estimation is only focused on these points. To maintain a required level of precision, it is suggested to use at least 1 knot for every 10 individuals (e.g., 100 knots for a dataset with 1000 individuals).

As with previous approaches, the accompanying web page (https://github.com/andreabellavia/statsmixtures) includes all code to replicate the results presented in this chapter using the NHANES simulated dataset.

5.2.6 Recent Extensions of the BKMR Framework

The original paper introducing BKMR only allowed evaluating continuous (normally distributed) outcomes. The approach has been later extended to estimate mixture-response associations in the presence of binary outcomes [12]. This extension is based on the concepts of GLM, but a probit rather than a logistic regression is used for computational efficiency. Doming-Relloso et al. [19] have also described how to extend the probit model to the analysis of time-to-event outcomes. Another extension of the original framework, fully integrated within the software, is the possibility of assessing clustered outcome data [12].

Additional extensions of the approach that could be of interest in several settings also include a longitudinal version of BKMR based on lagged regression, which can be used to evaluate time-varying mixture exposures [60, 100]. While this method is not yet implemented in the R package, it is useful to note that similar results can be achieved by evaluating time-varying effects through hierarchical selection. Specifically, multiple measurements of exposures can be included simultaneously in the kernel, grouping exposures by time. An example of this application can be found in Tyagi et al. [92], evaluating exposure to phthalates during pregnancy, measured at different trimester, as they relate to final gestational weight. By providing a measure of group importance, group PIPs can here be interpreted as measures of relative importance of the time windows of interest, thus allowing a better understanding of the timing of higher susceptibility to the exposure.

A recent work with high potential has attempted to unify the BKMR framework of response-surface estimation with the framework of exposure-indexing approaches, based on WQS. This unified framework, named Bayesian Multiple Index Model (BMIM), has the goal of facilitating interpretation of exposure weights within a Bayesian framework while incorporating non-linear relationships between index and outcome as well as non-additive relationships, all embedded within a variable selection framework [2, 66, 67]. At the time of this writing, applications of this approach are still sparse, and validation of this novel methodology in multiple contexts is required to better appreciate its advantages and limitations.

5.2.7 BKMR: Concluding Remarks

BKMR has rapidly become one of the most popular approaches for environmental mixtures, and the original manuscript has been cited over 1000 times in the 10 years since its publication. Applications of the approach have also been presented in other fields of epidemiology beyond the analysis of environmental exposures [6, 56]. Within environmental epidemiology, successful applications of BKMR have been conducted in several settings including mixtures of metals [7, 49, 97], air pollution [29, 55], endocrine-disrupting chemicals [10, 50, 88], and persistent chemicals [22, 98, 103].

In practice, applications of BKMR are often accompanied by other approaches and often used to assess whether previous results (e.g., regression-based, WQS) are affected by linearity and additivity assumptions. A potential problem when solely relying on BKMR for results presentation is that the nonparametric nature of the approach will generally limit the results to a qualitative assessment of non-linear and non-additive effects. As such, even in the presence of complex associations, it is recommended to validate results with alternative approaches like the ones discussed in the next subsection (see, e.g., results presentation in Zheng et al. [104]). In simple settings with a limited number of exposures and mostly linear associations, the flexibility of BKMR might not provide considerable advantages and only complicate the interpretability of results as compared to regression-based approaches. For example, the application of BKMR in the illustrative example used throughout this book, which includes simulated data with no interactions or non-linearity, does not provide any additional substantial insights as compared to previous methods. Nevertheless, if the real associations were unknown, this would be the first analytical step where additivity and non-linearity were confirmed from the data rather than assumed by the models.

Moreover, it is important to remember that model results, including the estimates of PIPs, are sensitive to the choice of the prior distributions. Even when these are kept non-informative, it is important to interpret PIPs as a relative measure of importance (as ranking the importance of exposures). The BKMR algorithm is more stable when it isn't dealing with exposures on vastly different scales. Because of that, standardizing exposures is good practice. Similarly, one should be wary of exposure outliers, and log-transforming exposures can also be considered.

Finally, it is important to mention that fitting a BKMR model is a computationally intensive procedure. In practice, application of BKMR on considerably large datasets might remain challenging even when using knots as previously described, and alternative approaches might be preferred in high-dimensional settings.

5.3 Generalized Additive Models (GAMs) and Their Extensions

5.3.1 Introduction

GAMs are extensions of the GLM framework where smooth functions are used to model covariates in place of the standard linear relationship [39, 102]. Applications of GAM are ubiquitous in clinical and epidemiological research, and its properties and flexibility have been long appreciated in environmental epidemiology [46, 87].

GAMs can be practically described as a direct attempt to relax linearity assumptions in regression modeling. Specifically, the outcome of interest is regressed on a sum of nonparametric smoothing functions, commonly based on spline modeling. For example, in a simple setting with two covariates of interest, we would fit the following model:

$$Y_i = s_1(X_1) + s_2(X_2) + \beta c_i + \epsilon_i, \tag{5.5}$$

where s_1 and s_2 are the specific nonparametric smooth functions used to relax linearity assumptions for X_1 and X_2, respectively.

This basic formulation of GAMs is estimated via maximum likelihood, and it can also be adapted to censored outcomes. Interactions can also be incorporated and smoothly estimated [82]. For example, we could integrate a smooth non-linear interaction in the previous model as

$$Y_i = s_1(X_1) + s_2(X_2) + s_3(X_1 \cdot X_2) + \beta c_i + \epsilon_i \tag{5.6}$$

As with any regression-based approach, this formulation of the model is subject to all limitations described in Sect. 3.2 and Sect. 5.1.3. In particular, adding smooth transformations for several variables will quickly lead to potential overfitting as the number of covariates increases. Not only we are including more variables and potential interaction terms, but we are also allowing for potential non-linear effect for each newly included variable. GAMs address this potential overfitting with penalization, in a similar fashion as the one described for Ridge regression. Penalty factors are only introduced for the smooth terms, resulting in a shrinkage procedure that makes functional forms less wiggly but that does not result in removing covariates for the model.

One of the advantages of GAM modeling is that, despite the nonparametric smoothing applied to each exposure-outcome association, common measures of variability and model performances from GLM can be computed, including R-squared and likelihood ratio test. Measures of variability are also available and confidence intervals can be derived [64]. P-values for the smooth terms can be computed as described in Wood et al. [101].

Table 5.3 Approximate p-values for smoothed terms in a GAM model without and with variable selection in the NHANES dataset

	p-value (w/o var. selection)	p-value (with var selection)
s(X_1)	0.036	0.020
s(X_2)	0.119	0.031
s(X_3)	0.330	0.100
s(X_4)	0.312	0.118
s(X_5)	0.950	0.911
s(X_6)	0.185	0.010
s(X_7)	0.698	0.954
s(X_8)	0.558	0.215
s(X_9)	0.599	0.438
s(X_{10})	0.177	0.002
s(X_{11})	0.565	0.299
s(X_{12})	0.154	0.041
s(X_{13})	0.018	0.005
s(X_{14})	0.322	0.062

5.3.2 GAM with Variable Selection

In more complex settings, such as the ones of environmental mixtures with several covariates potentially operating in a non-linear and non-additive fashion, the flexibility of GAM might not be enough to counterbalance its risk of data overfitting. The first column of Table 5.3 includes p-values for the smooth terms estimated by fitting a GAM model with standard penalization (i.e., without variable selection) in the NHANES data. This model fails to capture the most important predictors (X_6 and X_{12}) and rather provides the highest significance to X_{13}, which is correlated with X_{12}.

In these situations, extensions of GAM that operate variable selections should be considered. These extensions rely on modifying the penalty so that covariates can be excluded from the model. Two approaches for this penalty modification have been presented: GAM with a double penalty (GAMDP) and GAM with thin plate shrinkage smoother (GAMTS). Technical details of the two approaches can be found in Marra et al. [63], who suggested that GAMDP might work slightly better than GAMTS. Both options are fully implemented in the R package `mgcv` [102].

Results from the double penalty approach on the NHANES dataset are presented in the second column of Table 5.3 to allow direct comparison with the previous model without variable selection. This model is now able to detect both X_6 and X_{12} as relevant predictors in the exposure-outcome association.[5]

[5] Note that p-values do not have to be 0 for the variables to be removed. In this example, the procedure is eventually excluding $X_5, X_7, X_8, X_9, X_{11}$.

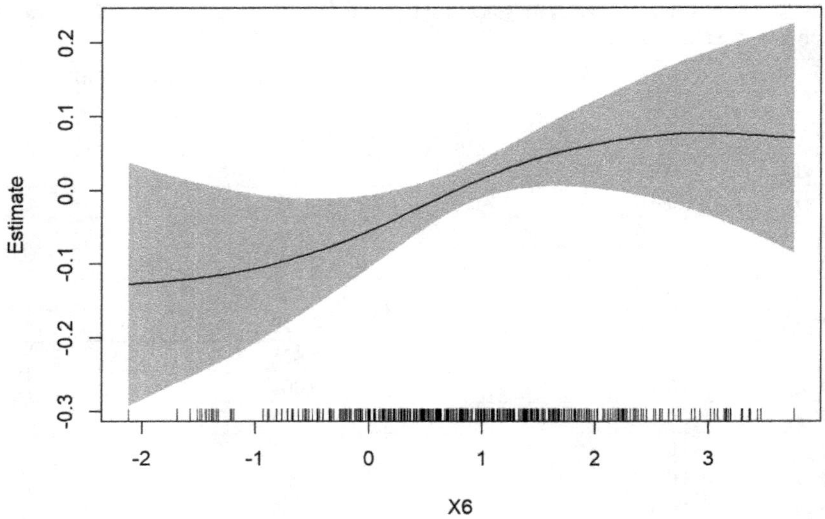

Fig. 5.10 Exposure-response function for X_6 (NHANES dataset) estimated from a generalized additive model with variable selection

As for BKMR, a graphical presentation of the exposure-response associations is required to fully understand the results. Figure 5.10, for example, shows the association between X_6 and the outcome in the NHANES data, estimated from a GAM with variable selection. The figure looks similar to the exposure-response function estimated by BKMR (Fig. 5.4). If smooth interactions were also included, bivariate response could also be plotted using the R package `visreg` [14].

5.3.3 Bayesian Approaches for Penalized GAM

The GAM framework has been further extended and generalized. In particular, Bayesian versions of penalized splines have proved successful in several applications [20]. Recent work has discussed the specific advantages of one of these Bayesian formulations—namely, Bayesian structured additive regression with spike-slab priors (BSTARSS)—in the context of environmental mixtures [52, 54]. BSTARSS might provide considerable advantages in complex settings as it allows formulating priors for penalized regression with variable selection that can cover both exposure-specific terms and parameters related to exposure groupings. BSTARSS is available in the R package `spikeSlabGAM` [85].

5.3.4 GAM: Concluding Remarks

GAMs provide a flexible tool to relax linearity assumptions embedded within the common framework of GLM. This methodological tool has been often applied for the assessment of environmental mixtures (see, e.g., [17, 18]), and some studies have shown that even the basic GAM formulation can successfully and comprehensively describe mixture-outcome associations in settings with limited complexity [104]. Often, GAM is used as a preliminary check to investigate potential non-linear associations that are then included in following analytical approaches [53].

Despite the presence of a penalization procedure that limits overfitting, the GLM-based nature of the framework makes GAM applications potentially subject to additional limitations. Collinearity, for example, will have greater effects on GAM results as compared to nonparametric models such as BKMR. In both cases, since the target is to investigate non-linear associations, graphical presentations will be required to comprehensively summarize results. Moreover, GAM and its extensions do not incorporate a straightforward estimation procedure for the cumulative mixture effect.

Complex settings with several covariates require double penalty procedures for a robust implementation of GAM, and improved performances in this context are provided by application of Bayesian approaches. A recent extensive simulation study on methods for complex non-linear correlated exposures has shown similar performances of BKMR, BSTARSS, GAMDP, and GAMST [54]. Applications of BKMR currently surpass applications of flexible GAM approaches, making BKMR—at this time—the standard and more natural choice to model environmental mixtures in the presence of potentially complex non-linear relationships. It is however recommended to explore these alternative approaches to fully exploit their advantages and identify those settings where each approach should be preferred.

5.4 Machine Learning for Environmental Mixtures

The application of ML approaches to the analysis of environmental mixtures is a field of very recent development that has been met with diverse levels of enthusiasm by the community [86]. The goal of this section is to simply outline some research areas in mixture analysis where ML could provide some advantages, describing some general concepts of the most common methods, and providing references of several recent applications of ML in environmental mixtures. In the final subsection, we will outline some of the challenges involved in the application and interpretation of ML in this context. References to technical papers are provided for readers interested in additional details of the discussed approaches.

5.4.1 General Overview of Machine Learning Approaches

An intuitive way of introducing the idea of ML, and how it differs from the statistical frameworks discussed so far, is by using the concept of the "two cultures" introduced by Breiman in his seminal 2001 paper [16]. One culture (statistics) assumes that data is generated by a given stochastic data model. The other culture (ML) uses algorithmic models and treats the data mechanisms as unknown. Using this classification, the distinction is not between different statistical approaches but rather between different ways of dealing with assumptions. A linear regression model, for example, makes the assumption that the data generating mechanism is subject to linearity and additivity. Under this point of view, we can already think of the approaches presented in the previous sections as attempts to bridge this gap between regression and ML. By using splines, for example, we are not making any assumption on the mechanistic nature of the functional form relating exposure and outcome, but we are rather letting the data inform us on the shape of this functional form.

As already discussed, relaxing assumptions comes with a risk of data overfitting, and this risk will be higher as the number of included covariates increases. ML algorithms, which provide a completely assumption-free framework, require robust and detailed tools to address overfitting. A key tool in this context is *cross-validation* [15]. The basic idea of cross-validation (CV) is to split the dataset into a number k of groups (commonly 10) and iteratively repeat a procedure where the model of interest is fit into $k-1$ groups and validated in the remaining group (k-fold CV). With ten groups, we would repeat the procedure ten times until each group has been used as a validation set, and final results would be averaged over these validation sets. CV is ubiquitous in ML. We have already encountered CV in Sect. 3.3 as a tool to identify the optimal level of λ in penalized regression. For this reason, penalized regressions such as LASSO and Elastic Net are sometimes referred to as semi-ML approaches [25]. Broadly speaking, ML approaches include CV at two different phases. In a first layer, CV is used to identify the optimal value of some specific *hyperparameters*, which can be thought of as external configuration variables used by the human to tune the machine [75]. This phase of hyperparameters tuning, which is generally conducted in a training dataset, is followed by the model estimation in the validation setting, where CV is also used for model building and performance evaluation.

The vast majority of ML approaches of interest in the context of environmental epidemiology are based on the concept of tree-based recursive partitioning [90]. This idea was first applied in the development of *classification and regression trees* (CART) [30, 77], which remain to this day a valuable tool in several contexts. Bayesian versions of CART have also been presented [45]. The concepts of CART were then extended to the generalization of several *ensemble methods*, where the goal is to improve the accuracy of results from a CART model by combining several models rather than using only one. In particular, the general framework of *random forests* [15, 41] provides considerable advantages in this aggregation procedure and has become one of the most popular ML approaches. More recently, *gradient boosting* has been presented as an alternative ensemble approach that can also take into account errors of previous trees in the build-up of a subsequent tree [23]. Boosting has been defined as "one of the most powerful learning ideas introduced" [40], and its applications have been extremely successful in several fields including clinical and epidemiologic research.

5.4.2 Areas of Interest in the Analysis of Environmental Mixtures

There are several reasons why ML approaches might be appealing to researchers interested in environmental mixtures, as documented by the increasing number of applications in the literature.

Interaction Testing
Section 5.1 motivated the importance of accounting for non-additive effects in mixtures research and underlined that interactions could be defined at increasing levels of complexity. For example, in a setting with three exposures, we could define up to three levels: (i) the main effects; (ii) all pairs of two-way interactions, and (iii) a three-way interaction. Increasing the number of exposures also increases the order of interaction testing one might want to conduct. The methods discussed in Sects. 5.2 and 5.3 represent powerful tools for the detection of non-linear associations, but several questions on interactions are still left unaddressed. GAM requires pre-specification of interactions in the model. BKMR accounts for higher-order interaction in a nonparametric fashion, but only provides graphical tools for a qualitative assessment of potential low-order interactions [1]. These results can be used for hypothesis generation and as a preliminary screening tool, but more robust approaches are required for those settings where interactions are of high interest [48].

ML approaches allow integrating high-order interactions without any assumption or pre-specification, all embedded within a CV procedure that can address overfitting. In particular, approaches based on random forests and gradient boosting can be particularly useful as one of their hyperparameters[6] has a direct interpretation in terms of orders of interactions [9]. Several applications of ML approaches for the detection of complex interactions in environmental mixtures have been presented and discussed. Sun et al. [91] and Barrera et al. [5] provided systematic comparisons of different approaches when interaction assessment is the main research question. The most common approaches used in applied research include random forests (see, e.g., [76]), boosting methods (e.g., [51, 58, 61, 72]), and Bayesian approaches

[6] Specifically, the hyperparameter "depth".

(e.g., [21, 69, 83]). Recent work also discussed ML within the framework of environmental risk score [73] and WQS [68] for interaction assessment.

Patterns Identification
Without formally defining them as such, we had already discussed some ML approaches in Chap. 2. The distinction we introduced between supervised and unsupervised approaches was in fact introduced in the context of ML to differentiate between methods that take or do not take the outcome into account. Unsupervised approaches such as cluster analysis, which uses data-driven techniques to group individuals, have been widely used in several fields as a powerful ML approach for patterns identification [42]. Formal applications of cluster analysis, PCA, as well as other unsupervised learning approaches are commonly used in mixture analyses where complex data require robust assessment of individuals' similarity or data reduction [3, 8, 27, 28, 57, 78].

Exposome-Wide Research
A final major topic where ML is receiving increasing attention in environmental epidemiology is for those settings where a high-dimensional number of predictors are jointly evaluated within an exposome-wide approach [47, 62, 71, 79]. In this context, the environmental mixture of interest might encompass chemicals and pollutants from different families and sources, often integrated with additional covariates such as occupational exposures, medications, or behavioral factors. ML is used here to accommodate the increasing complexity that addressing the exposome as a whole introduces [11, 95, 96]. A common analytical procedure in this context is to proceed in a two-stage fashion, using ML for a preliminary screening of covariates or interactions that are later included in a regression-based approach [91].[7]

5.4.3 Machine Learning: Concluding Remarks

Technical instruments to assess more detailed individual exposures within the exposome framework are becoming more readily available, resulting in larger and more complex data available for analyses in environmental epidemiology studies. In this context, it is natural to expect that more researchers will be interested in exploiting the potential advantages of ML. Despite the use of ML in environmental mixtures research is still in its embryonic phase, some general considerations can already be made. First, the advantages and flexibility of ML often come with a drawback in terms of results interpretation. Common tools that are very familiar to epidemiologists and public health practitioners, such as beta coefficients, confidence intervals, or p-values, together with classical measures of associations

[7] As discussed in Sect. 3.3.5, careful interpretations of p-values and standard errors should be reported when using this two-stage approach.

such as odds ratios and hazard ratios, will not be available when using ML.[8] The topic of *interpretable machine learning* is therefore of primary importance, and the discussion on the extent to which ML can provide interpretable results in environmental mixture analysis is an ongoing topic [26, 68, 70, 86]. In this context, a key factor to take into account is the ability of the chosen statistical approach to detect causal factors within the mixture rather than signals of associations. Concepts of causality in mixtures research are key to translate results into potential policies and/or public health recommendations, and will be further discussed in the next chapter.

References

1. Joseph Antonelli, Maitreyi Mazumdar, David Bellinger, David Christiani, Robert Wright, and Brent Coull. Estimating the health effects of environmental mixtures using bayesian semiparametric regression and sparsity inducing priors. 2020.
2. Joseph Antonelli, Ander Wilson, and Brent A Coull. Multiple exposure distributed lag models with variable selection. *Biostatistics*, 25(1):1–19, 2024.
3. Elena Austin, Brent Coull, Dylan Thomas, and Petros Koutrakis. A framework for identifying distinct multipollutant profiles in air pollution data. *Environment international*, 45:112–121, 2012.
4. Sudipto Banerjee, Alan E Gelfand, Andrew O Finley, and Huiyan Sang. Gaussian predictive process models for large spatial data sets. *Journal of the Royal Statistical Society Series B: Statistical Methodology*, 70(4):825–848, 2008.
5. Jose Barrera-Gómez, Lydiane Agier, Lützen Portengen, Marc Chadeau-Hyam, Lise Giorgis-Allemand, Valérie Siroux, Oliver Robinson, Jelle Vlaanderen, Juan R González, Mark Nieuwenhuijsen, et al. A systematic comparison of statistical methods to detect interactions in exposome-health associations. *Environmental Health*, 16:1–13, 2017.
6. Jemar R Bather, Taylor J Robinson, and Melody S Goodman. Bayesian kernel machine regression for social epidemiologic research. *Epidemiology*, pages 10–1097.
7. Julia A Bauer, Katrina L Devick, Jennifer F Bobb, Brent A Coull, David Bellinger, Chiara Benedetti, Giuseppa Cagna, Chiara Fedrighi, Stefano Guazzetti, Manuela Oppini, et al. Associations of a metal mixture measured in multiple biomarkers with iq: evidence from italian adolescents living near ferroalloy industry. *Environmental health perspectives*, 128(9):097002, 2020.
8. Liza-Marie Beckers, Werner Brack, Janek Paul Dann, Martin Krauss, Erik Müller, and Tobias Schulze. Unraveling longitudinal pollution patterns of organic micropollutants in a river by non-target screening and cluster analysis. *Science of the Total Environment*, 727:138388, 2020.
9. Andrea Bellavia, Aisha S Dickerson, Ran S Rotem, Johnni Hansen, Ole Gredal, and Marc G Weisskopf. Joint and interactive effects between health comorbidities and environmental exposures in predicting amyotrophic lateral sclerosis. *International journal of hygiene and environmental health*, 231:113655, 2021.

[8] These common measures and tools, nevertheless, are not exempt to challenging interpretation themselves. See for example issues with p-values and confidence intervals [37], hazard ratios [43], and odds ratios [74].

10. Andrea Bellavia, Runyu Zou, Richelle D Björvang, Kristine Roos, Ylva Sjunnesson, Ida Hallberg, Jan Holte, Anne Pikki, Virissa Lenters, Lützen Portengen, et al. Association between chemical mixtures and female fertility in women undergoing assisted reproduction in sweden and estonia. *Environmental research*, 216:114447, 2023.
11. Joline WJ Beulens, Maria GM Pinho, Taymara C Abreu, Nicole R den Braver, Thao M Lam, Anke Huss, Jelle Vlaanderen, Tabea Sonnenschein, Noreen Z Siddiqui, Zhendong Yuan, et al. Environmental risk factors of type 2 diabetes—an exposome approach. *Diabetologia*, 65(2):263–274, 2022.
12. Jennifer F Bobb, Birgit Claus Henn, Linda Valeri, and Brent A Coull. Statistical software for analyzing the health effects of multiple concurrent exposures via bayesian kernel machine regression. *Environmental Health*, 17(1):1–10, 2018.
13. Jennifer F Bobb, Linda Valeri, Birgit Claus Henn, David C Christiani, Robert O Wright, Maitreyi Mazumdar, John J Godleski, and Brent A Coull. Bayesian kernel machine regression for estimating the health effects of multi-pollutant mixtures. *Biostatistics*, 16(3):493–508, 2015.
14. Patrick Breheny and Woodrow Burchett. Visualization of regression models using visreg. *The R Journal*, 9(2):56–71, 2017.
15. Leo Breiman. Random forests. *Machine learning*, 45:5–32, 2001.
16. Leo Breiman. Statistical modeling: The two cultures (with comments and a rejoinder by the author). *Statistical science*, 16(3):199–231, 2001.
17. Maribel Casas, Damaskini Valvi, Ana Ballesteros-Gomez, Mireia Gascon, Mariana F Fernández, Raquel Garcia-Esteban, Carmen Iñiguez, David Martínez, Mario Murcia, Nuria Monfort, et al. Exposure to bisphenol a and phthalates during pregnancy and ultrasound measures of fetal growth in the inma-sabadell cohort. *Environmental health perspectives*, 124(4):521–528, 2016.
18. Birgit Claus Henn, David C Bellinger, Marianne R Hopkins, Brent A Coull, Adrienne S Ettinger, Rebecca Jim, Earl Hatley, David C Christiani, and Robert O Wright. Maternal and cord blood manganese concentrations and early childhood neurodevelopment among residents near a mining-impacted superfund site. *Environmental health perspectives*, 125(6):067020, 2017.
19. Arce Domingo-Relloso, Maria Grau-Perez, Laisa Briongos-Figuero, Jose L Gomez-Ariza, Tamara Garcia-Barrera, Antonio Dueñas-Laita, Jennifer F Bobb, F Javier Chaves, Marianthi-Anna Kioumourtzoglou, Ana Navas-Acien, et al. The association of urine metals and metal mixtures with cardiovascular incidence in an adult population from spain: the hortega follow-up study. *International journal of epidemiology*, 48(6):1839–1849, 2019.
20. Ludwig Fahrmeir, Thomas Kneib, and Stefan Lang. Penalized structured additive regression for space-time data: a bayesian perspective. *Statistica Sinica*, pages 731–761, 2004.
21. Federico Ferrari and David B Dunson. Bayesian factor analysis for inference on interactions. *Journal of the American Statistical Association*, 116(535):1521–1532, 2021.
22. Pauline Frenoy, Vittorio Perduca, German Cano-Sancho, Jean-Philippe Antignac, Gianluca Severi, and Francesca Romana Mancini. Application of two statistical approaches (bayesian kernel machine regression and principal component regression) to assess breast cancer risk in association to exposure to mixtures of brominated flame retardants and per-and polyfluorinated alkylated substances in the e3n cohort. *Environmental Health*, 21(1):27, 2022.
23. Jerome H Friedman. Greedy function approximation: a gradient boosting machine. *Annals of statistics*, pages 1189–1232, 2001.
24. Chris Gennings, Walter H Carter, Julie A Campain, Dong-soon Bae, and Raymond SH Yang. Statistical analysis of interactive cytotoxicity in human epidermal keratinocytes following exposure to a mixture of four metals. *Journal of Agricultural, Biological, and Environmental Statistics*, 7:58–73, 2002.
25. Thomas A Gerds and Michael W Kattan. *Medical risk prediction models: with ties to machine learning*. Chapman and Hall/CRC, 2021.

26. Elizabeth A Gibson, Jeff Goldsmith, and Marianthi-Anna Kioumourtzoglou. Complex mixtures, complex analyses: an emphasis on interpretable results. *Current environmental health reports*, 6:53–61, 2019.
27. Elizabeth A Gibson, Junhui Zhang, Jingkai Yan, Lawrence Chillrud, Jaime Benavides, Yanelli Nunez, Julie B Herbstman, Jeff Goldsmith, John Wright, and Marianthi-Anna Kioumourtzoglou. Principal component pursuit for pattern identification in environmental mixtures. *Environmental Health Perspectives*, 130(11):117008, 2022.
28. Elizabeth Atkeson Gibson. *Statistical and machine learning methods for pattern identification in environmental mixtures*. Columbia University, 2021.
29. Amanda J Goodrich, Michael J Kleeman, Daniel J Tancredi, Yunin J Ludeña, Deborah H Bennett, Irva Hertz-Picciotto, and Rebecca J Schmidt. Ultrafine particulate matter exposure during second year of life, but not before, associated with increased risk of autism spectrum disorder in bkmr mixtures model of multiple air pollutants. *Environmental Research*, 242:117624, 2024.
30. AD Gordon, L Breiman, JH Friedman, RA Olshen, and Cj J Stone. Classification and regression trees. *Biometrics*, 40(3):874, 1984.
31. Sander Greenland. Avoiding power loss associated with categorization and ordinal scores in dose-response and trend analysis. *Epidemiology*, 6(4):450–454, 1995.
32. Sander Greenland. Dose-response and trend analysis in epidemiology: alternatives to categorical analysis. *Epidemiology*, pages 356–365, 1995.
33. Sander Greenland. Bayesian perspectives for epidemiological research: I. foundations and basic methods. *International journal of epidemiology*, 35(3):765–775, 2006.
34. Sander Greenland. Smoothing observational data: a philosophy and implementation for the health sciences. *International statistical review*, 74(1):31–46, 2006.
35. Sander Greenland. Bayesian perspectives for epidemiological research. II. regression analysis. *International journal of epidemiology*, 36(1):195–202, 2007.
36. Sander Greenland. Bayesian perspectives for epidemiologic research: III. bias analysis via missing-data methods. *International journal of epidemiology*, 38(6):1662–1673, 2009.
37. Sander Greenland, Stephen J Senn, Kenneth J Rothman, John B Carlin, Charles Poole, Steven N Goodman, and Douglas G Altman. Statistical tests, p values, confidence intervals, and power: a guide to misinterpretations. *European journal of epidemiology*, 31(4):337–350, 2016.
38. Frank E. Harrell. *General Aspects of Fitting Regression Models*, pages 13–44. Springer International Publishing, Cham, 2015.
39. Trevor Hastie and Robert Tibshirani. Generalized additive models for medical research. *Statistical methods in medical research*, 4(3):187–196, 1995.
40. Trevor Hastie, Robert Tibshirani, Jerome Friedman, Trevor Hastie, Robert Tibshirani, and Jerome Friedman. Boosting and additive trees. *The elements of statistical learning: data mining, inference, and prediction*, pages 337–387, 2009.
41. Trevor Hastie, Robert Tibshirani, Jerome Friedman, Trevor Hastie, Robert Tibshirani, and Jerome Friedman. Random forests. *The elements of statistical learning: Data mining, inference, and prediction*, pages 587–604, 2009.
42. Trevor Hastie, Robert Tibshirani, Jerome Friedman, Trevor Hastie, Robert Tibshirani, and Jerome Friedman. Unsupervised learning. *The elements of statistical learning: Data mining, inference, and prediction*, pages 485–585, 2009.
43. Miguel A Hernán. The hazards of hazard ratios. *Epidemiology*, 21(1):13–15, 2010.
44. Kelly A Heys, Richard F Shore, M Glória Pereira, Kevin C Jones, and Francis L Martin. Risk assessment of environmental mixture effects. *RSC advances*, 6(53):47844–47857, 2016.
45. Jennifer Hill, Antonio Linero, and Jared Murray. Bayesian additive regression trees: A review and look forward. *Annual Review of Statistics and Its Application*, 7(1):251–278, 2020.
46. Jalila Jbilou and Salaheddine El Adlouni. Generalized additive models in environmental health: a literature review. *Novel approaches and their applications in risk assessment*, 120:2014–2016, 2012.

47. Daniel R Kowal, Mercedes Bravo, Henry Leong, Alexander Bui, Robert J Griffin, Katherine B Ensor, and Marie Lynn Miranda. Bayesian variable selection for understanding mixtures in environmental exposures. *Statistics in medicine*, 40(22):4850–4871, 2021.
48. Debamita Kundu, Sungduk Kim, Mary H Ward, and Paul S Albert. A comparison of statistical methods for studying interactions of chemical mixtures. *Statistics in Biosciences*, pages 1–17, 2024.
49. Allison Kupsco, Marianthi-Anna Kioumourtzoglou, Allan C Just, Chitra Amarasiriwardena, Guadalupe Estrada-Gutierrez, Alejandra Cantoral, Alison P Sanders, Joseph M Braun, Katherine Svensson, Kasey JM Brennan, et al. Prenatal metal concentrations and childhood cardiometabolic risk using bayesian kernel machine regression to assess mixture and interaction effects. *Epidemiology*, 30(2):263–273, 2019.
50. Allison Kupsco, Haotian Wu, Antonia M Calafat, Marianthi-Anna Kioumourtzoglou, Marcela Tamayo-Ortiz, Ivan Pantic, Alejandra Cantoral, Maricruz Tolentino, Emily Oken, Joseph M Braun, et al. Prenatal maternal phthalate exposures and child lipid and adipokine levels at age six: A study from the progress cohort of mexico city. *Environmental research*, 192:110341, 2021.
51. Erik Lampa, Lars Lind, P Monica Lind, and Anna Bornefalk-Hermansson. The identification of complex interactions in epidemiology and toxicology: a simulation study of boosted regression trees. *Environmental health*, 13:1–17, 2014.
52. Nina Lazarevic, Adrian G Barnett, Peter D Sly, Anna C Callan, Ania Stasinska, Jane S Heyworth, Andrea L Hinwood, and Luke D Knibbs. Prenatal exposure to mixtures of persistent environmental chemicals and fetal growth outcomes in western australia. *International Journal of Hygiene and Environmental Health*, 240:113899, 2022.
53. Nina Lazarevic, Adrian G Barnett, Peter D Sly, and Luke D Knibbs. Statistical methodology in studies of prenatal exposure to mixtures of endocrine-disrupting chemicals: a review of existing approaches and new alternatives. *Environmental health perspectives*, 127(2):026001, 2019.
54. Nina Lazarevic, Luke D Knibbs, Peter D Sly, and Adrian G Barnett. Performance of variable and function selection methods for estimating the nonlinear health effects of correlated chemical mixtures: A simulation study. *Statistics in Medicine*, 39(27):3947–3967, 2020.
55. Haomin Li, Wenying Deng, Raphael Small, Joel Schwartz, Jeremiah Liu, and Liuhua Shi. Health effects of air pollutant mixtures on overall mortality among the elderly population using bayesian kernel machine regression (bkmr). *Chemosphere*, 286:131566, 2022.
56. Ruiqiang Li, Wenqiang Zhan, Xin Huang, Limin Zhang, Yan Sun, Zechen Zhang, Wei Bao, and Yuxia Ma. Investigating associations between depressive symptoms and anti-/pro-inflammatory nutrients in an elderly population in northern china: a bayesian kernel machine regression approach. *Journal of Inflammation Research*, pages 5201–5213, 2021.
57. Eric N Liberda, Aleksandra M Zuk, David S Di, Robert J Moriarity, Ian D Martin, and Leonard JS Tsuji. Complex environmental contaminant mixtures and their associations with thyroid hormones using supervised and unsupervised machine learning techniques. *Environmental Advances*, 4:100054, 2021.
58. Lars Lind, Samira Salihovic, Erik Lampa, and P Monica Lind. Mixture effects of 30 environmental contaminants on incident metabolic syndrome—a prospective study. *Environment international*, 107:8–15, 2017.
59. Crystal Linkletter, Derek Bingham, Nicholas Hengartner, David Higdon, and Kenny Q Ye. Variable selection for gaussian process models in computer experiments. *Technometrics*, 48(4):478–490, 2006.
60. Shelley H Liu, Jennifer F Bobb, Kyu Ha Lee, Chris Gennings, Birgit Claus Henn, David Bellinger, Christine Austin, Lourdes Schnaas, Martha M Tellez-Rojo, Howard Hu, et al. Lagged kernel machine regression for identifying time windows of susceptibility to exposures of complex mixtures. *Biostatistics*, 19(3):325–341, 2018.
61. Li Luo, Laurie G Hudson, Johnnye Lewis, and Ji-Hyun Lee. Two-step approach for assessing the health effects of environmental chemical mixtures: application to simulated datasets and real data from the navajo birth cohort study. *Environmental Health*, 18:1–16, 2019.

62. Léa Maitre, Jean-Baptiste Guimbaud, Charline Warembourg, Nuria Güil-Oumrait, Paula Marcela Petrone, Marc Chadeau-Hyam, Martine Vrijheid, Xavier Basagaña, Juan R Gonzalez, Exposome Data Challenge Participant Consortium, et al. State-of-the-art methods for exposure-health studies: results from the exposome data challenge event. *Environment international*, 168:107422, 2022.
63. Giampiero Marra and Simon N Wood. Practical variable selection for generalized additive models. *Computational Statistics & Data Analysis*, 55(7):2372–2387, 2011.
64. Giampiero Marra and Simon N Wood. Coverage properties of confidence intervals for generalized additive model components. *Scandinavian Journal of Statistics*, 39(1):53–74, 2012.
65. Olwenn Martin, Martin Scholze, Sibylle Ermler, Joanne McPhie, Stephanie K Bopp, Aude Kienzler, Nikolaos Parissis, and Andreas Kortenkamp. Ten years of research on synergisms and antagonisms in chemical mixtures: A systematic review and quantitative reappraisal of mixture studies. *Environment international*, 146:106206, 2021.
66. Glen McGee, Ander Wilson, Brent A Coull, and Thomas F Webster. Incorporating biological knowledge in analyses of environmental mixtures and health. *Statistics in Medicine*, 42(17):3016–3031, 2023.
67. Glen McGee, Ander Wilson, Thomas F Webster, and Brent A Coull. Bayesian multiple index models for environmental mixtures. *Biometrics*, 79(1):462–474, 2023.
68. Vishal Midya and Chris Gennings. Detecting shape-based interactions among environmental chemicals using an ensemble of exposure-mixture regression and interpretable machine learning tools. *Statistics in Biosciences*, 16(2):395–415, 2024.
69. Daniel Mork and Ander Wilson. Estimating perinatal critical windows of susceptibility to environmental mixtures via structured bayesian regression tree pairs. *Biometrics*, 79(1):449–461, 2023.
70. Yanelli Nunez, Elizabeth A Gibson, Eva M Tanner, Chris Gennings, Brent A Coull, Jeff Goldsmith, and Marianthi-Anna Kioumourtzoglou. Reflection on modern methods: good practices for applied statistical learning in epidemiology. *International Journal of Epidemiology*, 50(2):685–693, 2021.
71. Haykanush Ohanyan, Lützen Portengen, Anke Huss, Eugenio Traini, Joline WJ Beulens, Gerard Hoek, Jeroen Lakerveld, and Roel Vermeulen. Machine learning approaches to characterize the obesogenic urban exposome. *Environment international*, 158:107015, 2022.
72. Youssef Oulhote, Brent Coull, Marie-Abele Bind, Frodi Debes, Flemming Nielsen, Ibon Tamayo, Pal Weihe, and Philippe Grandjean. Joint and independent neurotoxic effects of early life exposures to a chemical mixture: A multi-pollutant approach combining ensemble learning and g-computation. *Environmental Epidemiology*, 3(5):e063, 2019.
73. Sung Kyun Park, Zhangchen Zhao, and Bhramar Mukherjee. Construction of environmental risk score beyond standard linear models using machine learning methods: application to metal mixtures, oxidative stress and cardiovascular disease in nhanes. *Environmental Health*, 16:1–17, 2017.
74. Alexander Persoskie and Rebecca A Ferrer. A most odd ratio:: interpreting and describing odds ratios. *American Journal of Preventive Medicine*, 52(2):224–228, 2017.
75. Philipp Probst, Anne-Laure Boulesteix, and Bernd Bischl. Tunability: Importance of hyperparameters of machine learning algorithms. *Journal of Machine Learning Research*, 20(53):1–32, 2019.
76. Li-Tang Qin, Jun-Yao Zhang, Qiong-Yuan Nong, Hong-Hu Zeng, Yan-Peng Liang, Ling-Yun Mo, et al. Classification and regression machine learning models for predicting the combined toxicity and interactions of antibiotics and fungicides mixtures. *Environmental Pollution*, page 124565, 2024.
77. J. Ross Quinlan. Induction of decision trees. *Machine learning*, 1:81–106, 1986.
78. Weeberb J Requia, Brent A Coull, and Petros Koutrakis. Regional air pollution mixtures across the continental us. *Atmospheric environment*, 213:258–272, 2019.
79. Ran S Rotem, Andrea Bellavia, Sabrina Paganoni, and Marc G Weisskopf. Medication use and risk of amyotrophic lateral sclerosis: using machine learning for an exposome-wide screen of

a large clinical database. *Amyotrophic Lateral Sclerosis and Frontotemporal Degeneration*, 25(3–4):367–375, 2024.
80. Patrick Royston, Douglas G Altman, and Willi Sauerbrei. Dichotomizing continuous predictors in multiple regression: a bad idea. *Statistics in medicine*, 25(1):127–141, 2006.
81. Patrick Royston, Gareth Ambler, and Willi Sauerbrei. The use of fractional polynomials to model continuous risk variables in epidemiology. *International journal of epidemiology*, 28(5):964–974, 1999.
82. David Ruppert, Matt P Wand, and Raymond J Carroll. *Semiparametric regression*. Number 12. Cambridge university press, 2003.
83. Danilo A Sarti, Estevão B Prado, Alan N Inglis, Antônia AL Dos Santos, Catherine B Hurley, Rafael A Moral, and Andrew C Parnell. Bayesian additive regression trees for genotype by environment interaction models. *The Annals of Applied Statistics*, 17(3):1936–1957, 2023.
84. Terrance Savitsky, Marina Vannucci, and Naijun Sha. Variable selection for nonparametric gaussian process priors: Models and computational strategies. *Statistical science: a review journal of the Institute of Mathematical Statistics*, 26(1):130, 2011.
85. Fabian Scheipl. spikeslabgam: Bayesian variable selection, model choice and regularization for generalized additive mixed models in r. *Journal of Statistical Software*, 43(14):1–24, 2011.
86. Charles W Schmidt. Into the black box: what can machine learning offer environmental health research?, 2020.
87. Joel Schwartz. Assessing confounding, effect modification, and thresholds in the association between ambient particles and daily deaths. *Environmental health perspectives*, 108(6):563–568, 2000.
88. Irene Souter, Andrea Bellavia, Paige L Williams, TIM Korevaar, John D Meeker, Joseph M Braun, Ralph A de Poortere, Maarten A Broeren, Jennifer B Ford, Antonia M Calafat, et al. Urinary concentrations of phthalate metabolite mixtures in relation to serum biomarkers of thyroid function and autoimmunity among women from a fertility center. *Environmental health perspectives*, 128(6):067007, 2020.
89. David J Spurgeon, Oliver AH Jones, Jean-Lou CM Dorne, Claus Svendsen, Suresh Swain, and Stephen R Stürzenbaum. Systems toxicology approaches for understanding the joint effects of environmental chemical mixtures. *Science of the total environment*, 408(18):3725–3734, 2010.
90. Carolin Strobl, James Malley, and Gerhard Tutz. An introduction to recursive partitioning: rationale, application, and characteristics of classification and regression trees, bagging, and random forests. *Psychological methods*, 14(4):323, 2009.
91. Zhichao Sun, Yebin Tao, Shi Li, Kelly K Ferguson, John D Meeker, Sung Kyun Park, Stuart A Batterman, and Bhramar Mukherjee. Statistical strategies for constructing health risk models with multiple pollutants and their interactions: possible choices and comparisons. *Environmental Health*, 12:1–19, 2013.
92. Pooja Tyagi, Tamarra James-Todd, Lidia Mínguez-Alarcón, Jennifer B Ford, Myra Keller, John Petrozza, Antonia M Calafat, Russ Hauser, Paige L Williams, and Andrea Bellavia. Identifying windows of susceptibility to endocrine disrupting chemicals in relation to gestational weight gain among pregnant women attending a fertility clinic. *Environmental Research*, 194:110638, 2021.
93. Tyler J VanderWeele. On the distinction between interaction and effect modification. *Epidemiology*, 20(6):863–871, 2009.
94. Tyler J VanderWeele and Mirjam J Knol. A tutorial on interaction. *Epidemiologic methods*, 3(1):33–72, 2014.
95. Roel Vermeulen, Emma L Schymanski, Albert-László Barabási, and Gary W Miller. The exposome and health: Where chemistry meets biology. *Science*, 367(6476):392–396, 2020.
96. Jelle Vlaanderen, Kees De Hoogh, Gerard Hoek, Annette Peters, Nicole Probst-Hensch, Augustin Scalbert, Erik Melén, Cathryn Tonne, G Ardine De Wit, Marc Chadeau-Hyam, et al. Developing the building blocks to elucidate the impact of the urban exposome on cardiometabolic-pulmonary disease: The EU expanse project. *Environmental Epidemiology*, 5(4):e162, 2021.

97. Cuicui Wang, Zongli Xu, Xinye Qiu, Yaguang Wei, Adjani A Peralta, Mahdieh Danesh Yazdi, Tingfan Jin, Wenyuan Li, Allan Just, Jonathan Heiss, et al. Epigenome-wide dna methylation in leukocytes and toenail metals: The normative aging study. *Environmental research*, 217:114797, 2023.
98. Zifan Wang, Cuilin Zhang, Paige L Williams, Andrea Bellavia, Blair J Wylie, Michele R Hacker, Kurunthachalam Kannan, Michael S Bloom, Kelly J Hunt, Russ Hauser, et al. Polybrominated diphenyl ethers in early pregnancy and preterm birth: Findings from the nichd fetal growth studies. *International journal of hygiene and environmental health*, 243:113978, 2022.
99. Timothy L Wiemken and Robert R Kelley. Machine learning in epidemiology and health outcomes research. *Annu Rev Public Health*, 41(1):21–36, 2020.
100. Ander Wilson, Hsiao-Hsien Leon Hsu, Yueh-Hsiu Mathilda Chiu, Robert O Wright, Rosalind J Wright, and Brent A Coull. Kernel machine and distributed lag models for assessing windows of susceptibility to environmental mixtures in children's health studies. *The annals of applied statistics*, 16(2):1090, 2022.
101. Simon N Wood. On p-values for smooth components of an extended generalized additive model. *Biometrika*, 100(1):221–228, 2013.
102. Simon N Wood. *Generalized additive models: an introduction with R.* chapman and hall/CRC, 2017.
103. Mingyu Zhang, Sheryl L Rifas-Shiman, Izzuddin M Aris, Abby F Fleisch, Pi-I Debby Lin, Amy R Nichols, Emily Oken, and Marie-France Hivert. Associations of prenatal per-and polyfluoroalkyl substance (PFAS) exposures with offspring adiposity and body composition at 16–20 years of age: Project viva. *Environmental health perspectives*, 131(12):127002, 2023.
104. Yinnan Zheng, Pi-I Debby Lin, Paige L Williams, Marc G Weisskopf, Andres Cardenas, Sheryl L Rifas-Shiman, Robert O Wright, Chitra Amarasiriwardena, Birgit Claus Henn, Marie-France Hivert, et al. Early pregnancy essential and non-essential metal mixtures and gestational glucose concentrations in the 2nd trimester: Results from project viva. *Environment international*, 155:106690, 2021.

Chapter 6
Additional Topics and Final Remarks

6.1 Causal Effects of Environmental Mixtures

Chapters 3– 5 tackled the main topic of this book by describing statistical methods for assessing mixture-health associations in population-based studies. Additional considerations are required, however, to understand the extent to which reported associations describe the presence of *causal effects*. This additional step is critical for translating results into potential public health recommendations and regulatory policies, which represent the ultimate goal of environmental mixtures research as discussed in Chap. 1.

How to draw causal conclusions from population-based studies has been a major topic of research within the last decades, and important advancements have been made to identify effect definition and analytical assumptions for causal inference. Several novel methodologies have been developed, and pluralistic approaches that involve considerations at both phases of study design and statistical analysis can be adopted to reduce the potential harm of common epidemiological bias such as confounding or selection bias and improve the identification of causal effects [18, 32, 42]. In environmental epidemiology, several studies have extended general concepts in causal inference to incorporate specific challenges of environmental exposures, particularly focusing on the topic of air pollution studies [6, 9, 13, 40]. Dominici and Zigler [13], in particular, provide an excellent introduction to the topic of causality in air quality research, discussing how questions of causal inference should be considered from the phase of study design and stressing the importance of a clear definition of potential targets for interventions or policies to identify the optimal analytical approach.

While providing a solid basis for the study of causal effects of environmental mixtures, the complexity of the simultaneous assessment of multiple exposures requires additional scrutiny. To this date, regulatory policies are still largely

A. Bellavia, *Statistical Methods for Environmental Mixtures*, Society, Environment and Statistics, https://doi.org/10.1007/978-3-031-78987-8_6

designed to regulate one pollutant or chemical at the time, thus hampering the implementation of integrated policies and possibly resulting in uncertainties about the exact impact of regulations. For this reason, several researchers and governmental or private institutions are increasingly advocating for research efforts that could improve our understanding of the causal effects of environmental mixtures accounting for the complex exposure to high-dimensional data. A first step toward a better understanding of causal effects in environmental mixtures analysis has involved the application of existing regression-based approaches for causal inference. These include the use of *G-computation* for indexing methods, as discussed in Sect. 4.3.4 with quantile G-computation [21], as well as the application of multivariate extensions of the *propensity score* [24, 41].[1] Nevertheless, additional work has outlined further complexities that arise in the specific context of multiple environmental exposures [51]. Weisskopf et al. [48, 49], for example, discussed the issue of *bias amplification* when evaluating environmental mixtures, showing through several examples illustrated by DAGs how the joint assessment of multiple exposures in regression modeling can amplify, rather than reduce, confounding bias. A recent work of Antonelli et al. [2] has instead attempted to define critical concepts in causal inference, such as the assumptions of positivity required to assess causal effects, to the specific setting of air pollution mixtures. Finally, Samanta and Antonelli discussed issues related to false discovery control when applying approaches that operate variable selection for main exposures and interactions [37].

To this date, the discussion on causal effects for environmental mixtures has only touched the surface of its complexity and mostly focused on settings with mixtures of a limited number of exposures. As the dimensionality of the mixture increases, it becomes more important to carefully consider how the study design and the modeling assumptions affect the interpretability of the results from a causal perspective [16].

6.1.1 A Note on Confounding and Effect Modification

A multivariable regression model, in addition to mutually adjusting for all co-exposures of interest (e.g., the mixture components), often includes additional covariates that are required for confounding adjustment. The vast majority of approaches we have discussed throughout this book allow adjusting for potential confounders, thus providing a first step toward a better interpretation of associations as causal effects. When adjusting for additional covariates, however, it is important to remember that a certain variable could be both a confounder and an effect modifier (e.g., this is the case for Z_3 in the NHANES data). As described in Sect. 5.1.2, effect modification implies the presence of some level of interaction, which should

[1] For a gentle introduction to the concept of propensity score and its applications in causal inference, the reader can refer to the excellent introduction by Austin [3].

be incorporated for a correct model specification. Including interaction terms between mixture components and external covariates is not a straightforward procedure for most of the described methodologies. Nevertheless, *stratification* over levels of the effect modifier can be conducted for all approaches and is recommended to investigate whether the effect of the mixture or its components are modified over levels of external covariates (e.g., Z_3 in the NHANES dataset). Effect modification has critical interpretation within a causal inference framework for the identification of specific subgroups that would most benefit from potential interventions and recommendations [43].

6.2 Mediation Analysis to Assess the Role of Environmental Mixtures Within the Exposome

In Chap. 1 we introduced the *exposome* as a novel paradigm to define the complex system of exposures individuals are affected by throughout their lifetime [45]. The exposome involves the integration of several systems of exposures from environmental mixtures to social and lifestyle components that not only have a potential to independently affect human health but are also causally related within each other. Figure 6.1, for example, shows a potential causal pathway that relates modifiable sources of exposures (e.g., personal care products), a mixture of environmental chemicals (e.g., parabens), and a health outcome (e.g., diabetes).

In this example, the use of personal care products can increase the risk of diabetes either through causal pathways that involve the harmful effects of its chemical components or through other independent pathways. In this context it is usually of interest to disentangle the extent to which policy regulations to banning parabens would decrease the risk of diabetes associated with personal care products use. *Mediation analysis* is an established causal inference approach that provides

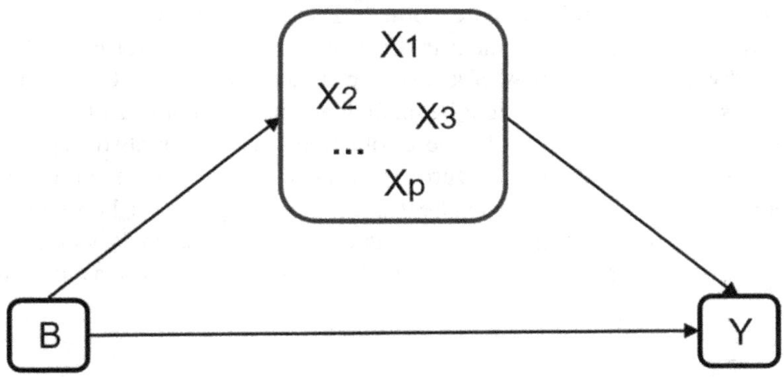

Fig. 6.1 Environmental mixture as a potential mediator of the effect of B on Y

a natural framework to address these questions. Specifically, mediation analysis allows decomposing the effect of the exposure (personal care products) on the outcome (diabetes) into pathways that involve the *mediator* (parabens) and independent pathways that operate through other mechanisms.[2] Approaches to integrate environmental mixtures as potential mediators in a mediation analysis framework include the application of methods for variable selection (e.g., LASSO, BKMR) to identify specific mediators of interest, or creating one or more mixture indices (e.g., WQS, PCA) to summarize the mixture into a few uncorrelated mediators [5]. Illustrations of these approaches in applied research include, among others, the study of metal mixtures as mediators of the association between socioeconomic status and health [35] and persistent chemicals as contributors to racial-ethnic disparities in preterm birth [47].

In addition to incorporating all external exposures, the exposome framework also attempts to integrate biological mechanisms (labeled *internal* exposome) that are involved in the processes leading from exposure to health. In this context, it might be of interest to assess an environmental mixture as the exposure in a mediation analysis model where internal exposome data (e.g., epigenetics) is evaluated as mediators of the health effects of environmental mixtures [7, 12]. Applications of mediation analysis in this setting have largely relied on extensions of BKMR [12, 46] and have been applied to a variety of topics including mixtures of metals [38], per- and polyfluoroalkyl (PFAS) substances [8], and air pollutants [23].

6.3 Incorporating Binary and Zero-Inflated Exposures

Throughout the presentation and discussion of the approaches described in this book, we have made an implicit assumption: components of an environmental mixture are described by *continuous* covariates. Section 2.2 discussed how the nature of environmental chemicals produces strictly positive and commonly skewed continuous covariates, and how standardization and log transformation can be used to make these variables look more normal. There are several settings, however, where even these operations remain ineffective. This happens, for example, when several individuals have values of a certain chemical under the LOD. Continuous imputations are available but might be inefficient when the number of non-detected samples is substantially high. In these situations, a more realistic approach is to either treat these values as a zero exposure or impute them with the same number (e.g., LOD/2 as discussed in Sect. 2.2). These imputations, however, disrupt the continuous nature of the covariate and might require analytical tools that allow treating the variable as binary, dichotomizing its values as detected vs

[2] A gentle and practical introduction to the concepts of mediation analysis can be found in Vanderweele [44]. The reader familiar with the general concepts and interested in additional details on the causal interpretation of mediation effects can instead refer to [29, 30, 39].

non-detected. This categorization has important analytical consequences as most of the methodologies we have described do not allow incorporating noncontinuous covariates within the mixture. Approaches for *zero-inflated* covariates exist [11] but have been rarely applied and studied in the context of environmental chemicals, where the tendency is to exclude such covariates from the mixture.

Similar considerations can be made when an exposome-wide approach is used to jointly evaluate environmental exposures and other dichotomous or categorical variables (e.g., medications, occupational exposures). This is one of those settings where machine learning approaches—which can incorporate several variables of different types including binary, categorical, and continuous—can become of particular interest [4, 31, 36].

6.4 General Overview of Recent Methodological Advancements

The rationale of this book was to provide a general yet comprehensive introduction to those analytical considerations and methodologies that could be regarded to as "established" within the field. As we'll discuss in the next (and final) section, the presented topics allow defining and conducting a solid analytical plan that can provide a robust understanding of mixture effects on health under several settings and levels of complexity. Nevertheless, the development and application of statistical approaches for environmental mixtures remains an active area of research. Novel methodologies and extensions of existing ones are in continuous development to address some specific challenges and considerations. Two specific publications provide an excellent overview to the reader interested in additional details of alternative approaches of recent development.

First, Joubert et al. [20] summarized the several advancements achieved by one of the major program initiatives of the US NIEHS, named "Powering Research through Innovative methods for Mixture in Epidemiology" (PRIME). Several of the recent extensions discussed in previous chapters (e.g., principal component pursuit, Bayesian Multiple Index Model) were funded through this initiative. Additional results of this program include, among others, the development of Bayesian approaches for complex data settings [14, 19, 22, 26, 33, 34] and methods for incorporating time-varying exposure effects [1, 15, 27, 28, 50].

Second, in 2021 the Barcelona Institute for Global Health (ISGlobal) held a data challenge event to compare existing approaches for the assessment of health effects in exposome-wide studies. Maitre et al. [25] provide an overview of the event conclusions, summarizing the results of 25 selected methods, and provide an excellent starting point to introduce the extensions and limitations of mixtures approaches for the more complex assessment of the exposome as a whole.

6.5 Final Remarks: Analyses Plans for Mixture Studies in Environmental Epidemiology

The goal of this primer was to discuss the challenges involved in the study of environmental mixtures as they relate to health outcomes in the population, and introduce the most common statistical approaches that can help addressing some of these challenges. The methods described should allow researchers to design and conduct a comprehensive analytical plan for assessing the health effects of environmental mixtures in several common data settings. This is a summary of the core points we discussed, with a set of final practical recommendations for the development of such analytical plans:

- Chemicals are found in the environment as mixtures and they affect human physiology through complex mechanisms. As such, assessing environmental factors as multiple combined exposures is required to fully understand their characteristics and health effects, and to correctly identify interventions, recommendations, and regulatory policies.
- To thoroughly study the health effects of environmental mixtures, several perspectives should be taken into account. The key research questions include:
  - Are there common patterns of exposures?
  - What is the overall (cumulative) mixture effect?
  - Who are the *bad actors* within the mixture?
  - Are there complex non-linear and non-additive effects that should be integrated?
- To address the complexity of exposure, it is strongly recommended to begin any analytical plan with unsupervised analysis, first assessing distributions and properties of individual chemicals (preprocessing) and then characterizing the mixture through the use of correlation analysis and dimensionality reduction techniques such as PCA. These phases provide critical information that will guide a better application and interpretation of subsequent analytical steps.
- Multivariable regression modeling should be included in any analytical plan, at least as a starting exploratory analysis.[3] This step provides an intuitive understanding on the level of data complexity to help guide the choice of what approach should follow. For example, extreme levels of collinearity, as indicated by extreme VIFs, might suggest the presence of complex clusters of exposures that most approaches will struggle to capture and identify, recommending the use of unsupervised summary scores (e.g., DEHP molar sum). Univariate models with spline transformations can also be used for a preliminary assessment of the potential presence of non-linear associations. It is nevertheless discouraged to include results from univariate assessments in the final set of results.

[3] With the notable exception of those high-dimensional settings where the number of mixture components surpasses the number of observations.

- After the preprocessing phase and mixture characterization, and in addition to multivariable regression, an ideal analytical plan should include the assessment of the overall effect, the identification of bad actors, and the estimation of their specific effects. Indexing approaches provide a suitable setting for estimating the overall effect of the mixture. Methods like WQS and quantile G-computation also estimate relative weights for each mixture component, thus providing an intuitive understanding of the potential bad actors contributing to the overall effect. However, it is important to remember that these methods, by summarizing the mixture with one or more indexes, only provide a ranking of mixture components and generally prevent the direct estimation of component-specific effects in the form of regression coefficients or graphical displays of exposure-response associations. To such end, variable selection methods such as penalized regression provide a complementary result that can be incorporated for a thorough assessment of the health effects of specific bad actors within the mixtures.
- Nonparametric approaches (e.g., BKMR) should be incorporated to assess whether results remain valid after relaxing assumptions of linearity and additivity. In general, results from these more complex methods should be reported as primary if the data is indeed complex enough to justify their application. In the presence of mostly linear and additive effects, regression-based and indexing approaches would likely provide robust results with an easier interpretation. Machine learning approaches should finally be considered with high-dimensional data, settings with specific interest in interaction assessment, and when integrating environmental mixtures within an exposome-wide perspective. It is critical, in these cases, to carefully consider the interpretability of results and their potential translation into public health messages.

Overall, the fundamental aspects of a successful analytical plan are:

- Clarifying the different research questions of interest
- Identifying data-specific challenges (e.g., high correlation, non-linearities, high number of non-detected values)
- Correctly choosing what classes of approaches allow addressing the specific questions of interest and inherent challenges
- Applying multiple approaches for results triangulation

Several applied papers can be used as a template of successful applications of this triangulation process (see, e.g., Cathey et al. [10] and Gibson et al. [17]).

6.5.1 Conclusion

In the introduction to this book, we stated that "*... One of the main reasons for this delayed transition to a multi-chemicals mindset [in environmental epidemiology] was certainly related to the analytical challenges that assessing complex* *environmental mixtures in population-based studies implicates."* At the time of this writing, this is not anymore a valid excuse. A substantial amount of research effort has been devoted to the clarification of such challenges and to the development of approaches that can address most of these complexities. While recognizing that several issues still have to be fully evaluated (see Sect. 6.4), it is now undeniable that environmental epidemiologists have the tools to assess complex mixtures of environmental exposures as they concretely occur, with the potential of providing a more realistic understanding of their health effects and a more targeted set of public health recommendations and interventions.

References

1. Joseph Antonelli, Ander Wilson, and Brent A Coull. Multiple exposure distributed lag models with variable selection. *Biostatistics*, 25(1):1–19, 2024.
2. Joseph Antonelli and Corwin M Zigler. Causal analysis of air pollution mixtures: Estimands, positivity, and extrapolation. *American Journal of Epidemiology*, page kwae115, 2024.
3. Peter C Austin. An introduction to propensity score methods for reducing the effects of confounding in observational studies. *Multivariate behavioral research*, 46(3):399–424, 2011.
4. Andrea Bellavia, Aisha S Dickerson, Ran S Rotem, Johnni Hansen, Ole Gredal, and Marc G Weisskopf. Joint and interactive effects between health comorbidities and environmental exposures in predicting amyotrophic lateral sclerosis. *International journal of hygiene and environmental health*, 231:113655, 2021.
5. Andrea Bellavia, Tamarra James-Todd, and Paige L Williams. Approaches for incorporating environmental mixtures as mediators in mediation analysis. *Environment international*, 123:368–374, 2019.
6. Marie-Abèle Bind. Causal modeling in environmental health. *Annual review of public health*, 40(1):23–43, 2019.
7. Michaël GB Blum, Linda Valeri, Olivier François, Solène Cadiou, Valérie Siroux, Johanna Lepeule, and Rémy Slama. Challenges raised by mediation analysis in a high-dimension setting. *Environmental health perspectives*, 128(5):055001, 2020.
8. Jessie P Buckley, Jordan R Kuiper, Bruce P Lanphear, Antonia M Calafat, Kim M Cecil, Aimin Chen, Yingying Xu, Kimberly Yolton, Heidi J Kalkwarf, and Joseph M Braun. Associations of maternal serum perfluoroalkyl substances concentrations with early adolescent bone mineral content and density: the health outcomes and measures of the environment (home) study. *Environmental health perspectives*, 129(9):097011, 2021.
9. Marco Carone, Francesca Dominici, and Lianne Sheppard. In pursuit of evidence in air pollution epidemiology: the role of causally driven data science. *Epidemiology*, 31(1):1–6, 2020.
10. Amber L Cathey, Deborah J Watkins, Zaira Y Rosario, Carmen Vélez, Bhramar Mukherjee, Akram N Alshawabkeh, José F Cordero, and John D Meeker. Biomarkers of exposure to phthalate mixtures and adverse birth outcomes in a puerto rico birth cohort. *Environmental health perspectives*, 130(3):037009, 2022.
11. Michelle L Dalrymple, Irene Lena Hudson, and Rodney PK Ford. Finite mixture, zero-inflated poisson and hurdle models with application to sids. *Computational Statistics & Data Analysis*, 41(3–4):491–504, 2003.
12. Katrina L Devick, Jennifer F Bobb, Maitreyi Mazumdar, Birgit Claus Henn, David C Bellinger, David C Christiani, Robert O Wright, Paige L Williams, Brent A Coull, and Linda Valeri. Bayesian kernel machine regression-causal mediation analysis. *arXiv preprint arXiv:1811.10453*, 2018.

13. Francesca Dominici and Corwin Zigler. Best practices for gauging evidence of causality in air pollution epidemiology. *American journal of epidemiology*, 186(12):1303–1309, 2017.
14. Federico Ferrari and David B Dunson. Bayesian factor analysis for inference on interactions. *Journal of the American Statistical Association*, 116(535):1521–1532, 2021.
15. Chris Gennings, Paul Curtin, Ghalib Bello, Robert Wright, Manish Arora, and Christine Austin. Lagged wqs regression for mixtures with many components. *Environmental research*, 186:109529, 2020.
16. Elizabeth A Gibson, Jeff Goldsmith, and Marianthi-Anna Kioumourtzoglou. Complex mixtures, complex analyses: an emphasis on interpretable results. *Current environmental health reports*, 6:53–61, 2019.
17. Elizabeth A Gibson, Yanelli Nunez, Ahlam Abuawad, Ami R Zota, Stefano Renzetti, Katrina L Devick, Chris Gennings, Jeff Goldsmith, Brent A Coull, and Marianthi-Anna Kioumourtzoglou. An overview of methods to address distinct research questions on environmental mixtures: an application to persistent organic pollutants and leukocyte telomere length. *Environmental Health*, 18:1–16, 2019.
18. Miguel A Hernán and James M Robins. Estimating causal effects from epidemiological data. *Journal of Epidemiology & Community Health*, 60(7):578–586, 2006.
19. Bora Jin, David B Dunson, Julia E Rager, David M Reif, Stephanie M Engel, and Amy H Herring. Bayesian matrix completion for hypothesis testing. *Journal of the Royal Statistical Society Series C: Applied Statistics*, 72(2):254–270, 2023.
20. Bonnie R Joubert, Marianthi-Anna Kioumourtzoglou, Toccara Chamberlain, Hua Yun Chen, Chris Gennings, Mary E Turyk, Marie Lynn Miranda, Thomas F Webster, Katherine B Ensor, David B Dunson, et al. Powering research through innovative methods for mixtures in epidemiology (prime) program: novel and expanded statistical methods. *International Journal of Environmental Research and Public Health*, 19(3):1378, 2022.
21. Alexander P Keil, Jessie P Buckley, Katie M O'Brien, Kelly K Ferguson, Shanshan Zhao, and Alexandra J White. A quantile-based g-computation approach to addressing the effects of exposure mixtures. *Environmental health perspectives*, 128(4):047004, 2020.
22. Daniel R Kowal. Fast, optimal, and targeted predictions using parameterized decision analysis. *Journal of the American Statistical Association*, 117(540):1875–1886, 2022.
23. Jessica E Laine, Barbara Bodinier, Oliver Robinson, Michelle Plusquin, Augustin Scalbert, Pekka Keski-Rahkonen, Nivonirina Robinot, Roel Vermeulen, Costanza Pizzi, Federica Asta, et al. Prenatal exposure to multiple air pollutants, mediating molecular mechanisms, and shifts in birthweight. *Environmental Science & Technology*, 54(22):14502–14513, 2020.
24. Kecheng Li, Tugba Akkaya-Hocagil, Richard J Cook, Louise M Ryan, R Colin Carter, Khue-Dung Dang, Joseph L Jacobson, and Sandra W Jacobson. Use of generalized propensity scores for assessing effects of multiple exposures. *Statistics in Biosciences*, 16(2):347–376, 2024.
25. Léa Maitre, Jean-Baptiste Guimbaud, Charline Warembourg, Nuria Güil-Oumrait, Paula Marcela Petrone, Marc Chadeau-Hyam, Martine Vrijheid, Xavier Basagaña, Juan R Gonzalez, Exposome Data Challenge Participant Consortium, et al. State-of-the-art methods for exposure-health studies: results from the exposome data challenge event. *Environment international*, 168:107422, 2022.
26. Kelly R Moran, David Dunson, Matthew W Wheeler, and Amy H Herring. Bayesian joint modeling of chemical structure and dose response curves. *The annals of applied statistics*, 15(3):1405, 2021.
27. Daniel Mork and Ander Wilson. Treed distributed lag nonlinear models. *Biostatistics*, 23(3):754–771, 2022.
28. Daniel Mork and Ander Wilson. Estimating perinatal critical windows of susceptibility to environmental mixtures via structured bayesian regression tree pairs. *Biometrics*, 79(1):449–461, 2023.
29. Ashley I Naimi, Jay S Kaufman, and Richard F MacLehose. Mediation misgivings: ambiguous clinical and public health interpretations of natural direct and indirect effects. *International journal of epidemiology*, 43(5):1656–1661, 2014.

30. Ashley I Naimi, Mireille E Schnitzer, Erica EM Moodie, and Lisa M Bodnar. Mediation analysis for health disparities research. *American journal of epidemiology*, 184(4):315–324, 2016.
31. Haykanush Ohanyan, Lützen Portengen, Anke Huss, Eugenio Traini, Joline WJ Beulens, Gerard Hoek, Jeroen Lakerveld, and Roel Vermeulen. Machine learning approaches to characterize the obesogenic urban exposome. *Environment international*, 158:107015, 2022.
32. Judea Pearl, Madelyn Glymour, and Nicholas P Jewell. *Causal inference in statistics: A primer*. John Wiley & Sons, 2016.
33. Michele Peruzzi, Sudipto Banerjee, David B Dunson, and Andrew O Finley. Grid-parametrize-split (grips) for improved scalable inference in spatial big data analysis. *arXiv preprint arXiv:2101.03579*, 2021.
34. Michele Peruzzi and David B Dunson. Spatial meshing for general bayesian multivariate models. *J. Mach. Learn. Res*, 25:1–49, 2024.
35. Juwel Rana, Stefano Renzetti, Rakibul Islam, Metodi Donev, Kai Hu, and Youssef Oulhote. Mediation effect of metal mixtures in the association between socioeconomic status and self-rated health among us adults: A weighted quantile sum mediation approach. *Exposure and Health*, 14(3):609–621, 2022.
36. Ran S Rotem, Andrea Bellavia, Sabrina Paganoni, and Marc G Weisskopf. Medication use and risk of amyotrophic lateral sclerosis: using machine learning for an exposome-wide screen of a large clinical database. *Amyotrophic Lateral Sclerosis and Frontotemporal Degeneration*, 25(3–4):367–375, 2024.
37. Srijata Samanta and Joseph Antonelli. Estimation and false discovery control for the analysis of environmental mixtures. *Biostatistics*, 23(4):1039–1055, 2022.
38. Samantha Schildroth, Linda Valeri, Katarzyna Kordas, Baoyi Shi, Alexa Friedman, Donald Smith, Donatella Placidi, Robert O Wright, Roberto G Lucchini, Roberta F White, et al. Assessing the mediating role of iron status on associations between an industry-relevant metal mixture and verbal learning and memory in italian adolescents. *Science of The Total Environment*, 906:167435, 2024.
39. Baoyi Shi, Christine Choirat, Brent A Coull, Tyler J VanderWeele, and Linda Valeri. Cmaverse: a suite of functions for reproducible causal mediation analyses. *Epidemiology*, 32(5):e20–e22, 2021.
40. Alice J Sommer, Emmanuelle Leray, Young Lee, and Marie-Abèle C Bind. Assessing environmental epidemiology questions in practice with a causal inference pipeline: An investigation of the air pollution-multiple sclerosis relapses relationship. *Statistics in Medicine*, 40(6):1321–1335, 2021.
41. Eugenio Traini, Anke Huss, Lützen Portengen, Matti Rookus, WM Monique Verschuren, Roel Vermeulen, and Andrea Bellavia. A multi-pollutant approach to estimate the causal effects of air pollution mixtures on overall mortality in a large prospective cohort of dutch individuals. 2021.
42. Jan P Vandenbroucke, Alex Broadbent, and Neil Pearce. Causality and causal inference in epidemiology: the need for a pluralistic approach. *International journal of epidemiology*, 45(6):1776–1786, 2016.
43. Tyler J VanderWeele. Confounding and effect modification: distribution and measure. *Epidemiologic methods*, 1(1):55–82, 2012.
44. Tyler J VanderWeele. Mediation analysis: a practitioner's guide. *Annual review of public health*, 37(1):17–32, 2016.
45. Roel Vermeulen, Emma L Schymanski, Albert-László Barabási, and Gary W Miller. The exposome and health: Where chemistry meets biology. *Science*, 367(6476):392–396, 2020.
46. A Wang, KL Devick, JF Bobbs, A Navas-Acien, BA Coull, and L Valeri. Bkmr-cma: A novel r command for mediation analysis in environmental mixture studies. In *ISEE Conference Abstracts*, volume 2020, 2020.

47. Zifan Wang, Cuilin Zhang, Paige L Williams, Andrea Bellavia, Blair J Wylie, Kurunthachalam Kannan, Michael S Bloom, Kelly J Hunt, and Tamarra James-Todd. Racial and ethnic disparities in preterm birth: a mediation analysis incorporating mixtures of polybrominated diphenyl ethers. *Frontiers in Reproductive Health*, 5:1285444, 2024.
48. Thomas F Webster and Marc G Weisskopf. Epidemiology of exposure to mixtures: we cant be casual about causality when using or testing methods. *arXiv preprint arXiv:2007.01370*, 2020.
49. Marc G Weisskopf, Ryan M Seals, and Thomas F Webster. Bias amplification in epidemiologic analysis of exposure to mixtures. *Environmental health perspectives*, 126(4):047003, 2018.
50. Ander Wilson, Hsiao-Hsien Leon Hsu, Yueh-Hsiu Mathilda Chiu, Robert O Wright, Rosalind J Wright, and Brent A Coull. Kernel machine and distributed lag models for assessing windows of susceptibility to environmental mixtures in children's health studies. *The annals of applied statistics*, 16(2):1090, 2022.
51. Corwin M Zigler. Invited commentary: the promise and pitfalls of causal inference with multivariate environmental exposures. *American Journal of Epidemiology*, 190(12):2658–2661, 2021.

www.ingramcontent.com/pod-product-compliance
Lightning Source LLC
Chambersburg PA
CBHW072043101025
33730CB00039B/19
* 9 7 8 3 0 3 1 7 8 9 8 6 1 *